PARKINSON'S EMPOWERMENT TRAINING

THE NEXT STEPS TOWARDS IMPROVING MOVEMENT, MEMORY, AND COGNITION

Table of Contents
Part One

Part Two

Inspiring Stories From:

Acknowledgements

Thank you to my clients, who have all taught me so much and inspired me greatly. You mean so much to me and I will always be here to help you to the best of my ability.

To Dr. Joseph Barry – a huge thank you for your belief in me and what I do to help our patients and clients.

Laura Olmos – thank you for your friendship and for being such a wonderful and positive influence on so many people. Thank you for your beautiful artwork. I am honored to have your artwork gracing the cover of my book.

To my dearest friend, the late Emily Gokey – thank you for working with and inspiring our clients. They loved working with you. You made a huge difference for all of them. We miss you terribly.

To Theresa and Elizabeth for being the best co-workers I could ever imagine working with.

Thank you to Stefan Sillner, Avrum Elmakis, Dr. Najeeb Thomas, Mike Hershkovitz, Eric Durak, Louis Lara, Martin Littlechild, Natalia Karbasova, Paul Peez, Rob Smith, Chris Fisher, and Jesse Ohliger for your support and belief in the work I do. I am grateful for your friendships!

Thank you to CLMBR, T2 Iso-Trainer, Power Plate, FitTech Club, BoBo Balance, Reaxing, Breath Belt, Rock Tape, Alpha Champs, Kayezen Vector, A-Champs, Vitruvian, Motion Guidance, Stick Mobility, ElectroSkip, FightCamp, Vivo Barefoot, Urban Poling, & StrongBoard Balance for your continued support and belief in what I do.

To my amazing family for always believing in me and for inspiring me so.

To my Godmother Teresa, Padre Amedeo, Father Prior, Sister Anne, and Peg Dolan for your friendship and spiritual guidance. You have all helped me more than you know. I am eternally grateful to all of you.

"Just get started and you'll get the energy to keep going" ~ *Karl Sterling*

Introduction

Thank you for investing in this book, my second book.

Unlike my first book, this book contains far less words from me, but very important information.

My number one goal *with this book is to succinctly deliver education that will help to better understand the workings of the brain and nervous systems, and how we can optimize neuroplasticity – and to explain it all as simply as possible.*

My second goal *is to offer intervention techniques and strategies that effectively transfer to activities of daily living to decrease fall risk and improve quality of movement and life for the person living with PD.*

My third goal is to MOTIVATE YOU. This book contains highly inspiring stories from

- *People living with Parkinson's*
- *Caregivers*
- *Doctors*
- *Movement Specialists*
- *Fitness Professionals*

If you read my first book, Parkinson's Regeneration Training, you probably learned a bit about Parkinson's disease, how it may affect a person, and intervention strategies to help slow disease progression and improve movement and quality of life.

As succinctly as possible, we will go deeper into many areas that were not thoroughly explored in book one, including:

- The job of the nervous system
- The many roles of dopamine

- Taking an in depth look at the process of neuroplasticity, how it varies between the young and the elderly, and how we can choose to maximize it
- Learning about other neurotransmitters and chemicals produced by the brain along with the role they play in neuroplasticity, cognition, movement, and functionality
- The many domains of cognition and memory
- Cognitive training concepts and exercises to help improve cognition and memory
- The eyes, vision, natural light and dark in relation to the circadian rhythm sleep-wake cycle
- The importance of sleep, mindfulness, and gratitude
- Benefits of music, art, self-expression, and being creative
- Nutrition in Parkinson's disease

This book is divided into two parts:

- Part one: the education and intervention strategies
- Part two: stories of inspiration written by people with Parkinson's, caregivers, trainers, and doctors.

As I always say during my workshops; much of what I teach is based on published research. But some of what I teach is not based on research. As practitioners, it is especially important that we do not get stuck inside

boundaries that prevent us from delivering effective intervention strategies to help our clients and patients. If we are not experimenting and thinking outside the box, we will not reach the potential we desire as practitioners.

More than anything, it is my goal to help you, the reader to gain a more comprehensive understanding of how we can help the person with Parkinson's to slow disease progression, manage disease symptoms, and improve quality of movement and life.

Best of all, the information in this book applies to ALL humans! We all have a brain and nervous systems. I use the concepts in this book with every person I work with, Parkinson's or not. I use these concepts during my own workouts. The results speak for themselves.

Are you ready to take a deeper look into all of this? I am, so let's go!

Part One

Parkinson's Education

Chapter 1

Hope

Belief

Empowerment

Never underestimate the power of HOPE!

Hope is defined as: desire accompanied by expectation of or belief in fulfillment.

Belief is defined as: trust, faith, or confidence in someone or something.

Empowerment is defined as: the process of becoming stronger or more confident, especially in controlling one's life and claiming one's rights.

Countless times in my work with people with Parkinson's around the world, I have observed little miracles that lead to major positive changes.

Example: a person with Parkinson's comes to an event hoping that something we teach will help them. As soon as they learn and execute a technique or strategy that helps them to regain or greatly improve an ability, BINGO! Their eyes light up with HOPE as they now see *possibility* because they *believe* in themselves.

It's as if a switch gets flipped *ON* and now, they're *empowered!* There's nothing like the feeling of empowerment. You see it in their eyes and their posture. You see it and feel it in their immediate change in energy. You see it in their movement.

And how about the ripple effect? This is huge. When someone realizes hope and feels empowered, people around them see it and feel it, too.

Hope can lead to empowerment and the feeling of being unstoppable. It can change lives.

It's the reason I keep researching, studying, and trying new things every single day. The more ways we can instill hope, real hope – the more we can help people to believe in themselves, feel empowered, and improve the quality of their lives - and a little hope can go a long way.

A gentleman with PD (Wayne) in Glenwood Springs, Colorado came to our workshop. At first, he was standoffish and angry, but he showed up and we were glad he joined us.

He told us that he hadn't been able to roll over without assistance in many years. So, we put mats on the floor, and everyone got down and laid on their backs.

Less than five minutes later, after teaching our simple, strategic rolling techniques, Wayne was easily rolling from back to front, and front to back in both directions. He learned how to leverage his body and easily propel himself in any direction when rolling.

You could see his energy change. In fact, he was smiling (something he hadn't yet done in our presence). He was no longer standoffish and angry. When he got up off the floor, his posture and gait improved. He was now unstoppable and for the rest of our two days together during the workshop, he was on fire and doing things he never thought he would do again.

Hope, belief, and empowerment have immeasurable value. This is only one of countless success stories. Let's move forward.

Chapter 2

The Brain & Nervous System

The subject of this chapter has filled entire libraries. In the interest of being succinct, I will be painting with a very broad brush and speaking in very general terms on the subject matter in this chapter.

I have studied the work of many great scientists and researchers. Dr. Andrew Huberman at Stanford University is among the most articulate of any scientist I know of.

This description of "the job of the nervous system" comes directly from Dr. Huberman (via many of his YouTube / podcast interviews). Let's take a look.

The nervous system includes two major branches: the central nervous system and the peripheral nervous system. Conceptually, these systems link the brain with the body and the body and all its organs with the brain.

Here is the step-by-step process:

We start with **sensation**:
- Our eyes allow us to see things
- Our nose allows us to sense smells
- Our ears allow us to hear sounds

- Our tongue allows us to taste
- Our skin can feel textures, heat, cold, stretch, and pressure.

We are sensing physical events all the time, many of which are subconscious.

Next, we have **perception**:
- The extent to which any one or more of these sensations become conscious, i.e., feet in contact with floor or shoe.
- Attention can de directed. If I ask, "how do your feet feel inside your shoes?" This sensation will likely remain subconscious until attention is directed to mindfully sensing how the feet feel. Once attention is directed, we perceive this sensation consciously.

After perception, we have **feelings / emotions**:

- The brain and body are designed to move us towards particular end goals. Feelings can drive us to these goals
- Feelings are mental experiences of body states. They signify physiological need (for example, hunger), tissue injury (for example, pain), optimal function (for example, well-being), threats to the organism (for example, fear or anger) or specific social interactions (for example, compassion, gratitude, or love). Feelings constitute a crucial component of the mechanisms of life regulation, from simple to complex. Their neural substrates can be found at all levels of the nervous system,

from individual neurons to subcortical nuclei and cortical regions. (Carvalho, 2013)

Next are **thoughts:**

Definition of *thought:*

- something that is <u>thought</u>: such as
  a: an individual act or product of thinking
  b: a developed <u>intention</u> or plan
  c: something (such as an opinion or belief) in the mind
  d: the intellectual product or the organized views and principles of a period, place, group, or individual (Merriam-Webster, n.d.)
- Thoughts may include memories and previous experiences
- Thoughts involve creating meaning out of perceptions

Lastly: **behaviours/actions:**

- Sensations, perceptions, feelings, and thoughts lead to our actions
- Behaviour is defined as:
  - the way in which someone conducts oneself or behaves
  - anything that an organism does involving action and response to stimulation
  - the response of an individual, group, or species to its environment
  - the way in which something functions or operates (Merriam-Webster, n.d.)

Entire books and graduate degree programs are devoted to the study of behaviour. I almost feel "wrong" in stopping here with my explanation of "the job of the nervous system." At the same time if you wish to learn more about any of this, jump onto www.*pubmed.ncbi.nlm.nih.gov* or Google Scholar and start searching. You will get endless amounts of information.

Meanwhile, we have now covered the primary steps involved in how the nervous system functions. This gives us enough knowledge to move forward.

Parkinson's Disease and the Nervous System - A Quick Review

We know that Parkinson's disease is a progressive nervous system disorder that affects movement. Symptoms start gradually, sometimes starting with a barely noticeable tremor in just one hand. Tremors are common, but the disorder also commonly causes stiffness or slowing of movement. (Clinic M. , Mayo Clinic, n.d.)

The immediate cause of PD is degeneration of brain cells on the area known as the substantia nigra, one of the movement control centers of the brain.

The degeneration of these brain cells causes a reduction in the production of dopamine (a chemical messenger responsible for transmitting signals between the substantia nigra to multiple brain regions and through the central and peripheral nervous systems).

Loss of dopamine results in greater difficulty producing smooth, intentional movements.

Let's take this a step further to gain a better understanding of how the job of the nervous system is relevant in all our movements and activities.

Interoception and Exteroception

While these have become buzz words of sorts lately, they are highly relevant with regards to our movement and activities of daily living.

Interoception is defined as the perception of sensations from inside the body and includes the perception of physical sensations related to internal organ function such as heartbeat, respiration, satiety, as well as the autonomic nervous system activity related to emotions. (Cynthia J. Price, 2018) Interoception can also be described as your perception of what is happening within your body.

Exteroception or exteroceptive body awareness (or "the body schema") refers to the implicit knowledge we have of our body in relation to space and movement. It results from the integration of multimodal exteroceptive signals (e.g., vision, sound, touch), vestibular and proprioceptive systems, and voluntary motor systems. Even though the term "body schema" is more commonly used, we refer to exteroceptive body awareness to highlight the relationship with interoceptive body awareness. (Camila Valenzuela-Moguillansky, 2017) Exteroception can also be described as our perception of what is happening in the outside world.

The nervous system is responsible for bridging interoception with exteroception using specific sets of neurons to match our inner world with the demands of the outside world. (Andrew Huberman, 2020)

For example, when we are sleeping, we are in complete interoception with no awareness of what is happening in the outside world. (Andrew Huberman, 2020)

And, perhaps you have been in this situation, as I have: you're running through an airport, trying to get to the gate before they shut the door. Your sole focus is making the

flight! Meanwhile, you are sweating, your heart rate is elevated, and you are breathing hard, but you are completely unaware of this until you stop running. You've been in a state of complete exteroception and solely focused on making it to the gate on time. (Andrew Huberman, 2020)

Most of the time, however – we are between interoception and exteroception, going back and forth. It is the job of the nervous system to keep us balanced between the two. (Andrew Huberman, 2020)

Parkinson's, Falls, and a Compromised Nervous System

Falling is our number one concern for the person living with PD. In fact, complications from a fall are the number one cause of mortality in the PD population.

Once a person falls, they enter the "faller" category and are much more likely to fall again (and again). Our goal? Keep the person with PD out of the faller category!

If we summarize everything up to this point in the book, we now know the job of the nervous system and that the person with Parkinson's is likely to experience challenges with movement and are at an increased risk of falls and injury.

What can we do?

To answer this question, we will start with a disclaimer as it is paramount that you realize:

- we are not claiming that we will stop or reverse Parkinson's disease
- we are not here with the intention of replacing medical experts, neurologists, or medications

- we are here to deliver effective intervention strategies and techniques to complement medications and medical therapies
- it is very likely (but not guaranteed) that if the person with PD puts our strategies into effect, they will slow disease progression, improve cognition, memory, gait, and movement

Chapter 3

Maximizing Neuroplasticity: A Two-Step Process

In Parkinson's disease, movement becomes compromised. And often-times, cognition and memory become compromised. So, how can we improve movement, cognition, and memory? The answer is: *by harnessing the power of neuroplasticity!*

We know that the brain has the amazing ability to develop new neural pathways which allows us to learn and develop new skills.

But how does this work exactly? The answer is: it is a *two-step process* for most of us.

From the time we are infants up until the age of approximately 25 years, the human brain is highly plastic and moldable. For infants and young children, mere exposure can be sufficient for learning.

Examples include:

- learning a language
- learning to walk
- feeding ourselves
- learning to read
- learning to play an instrument
- learning to ride a bicycle

and of course, there are countless other things I could list, but you get the idea.

During these early years, much less effort is required to learn (for most of us) compared to when we get older.

So, why is it more difficult to learn as we get older and CAN we still learn as we age? YES, we can, however after approximately age 25, the brain becomes less moldable and the process for learning changes and becomes a two-step process.

Even though learning generally becomes more work, we can optimize every learning event to get the most out of it.

This is highly relevant, especially when someone is dealing with a condition like Parkinson's disease, Alzheimer's, or any other neurological condition where areas of the brain are not functioning well or dying off.

The two-step process outlined in the following pages tells us exactly HOW to approach every learning event so we can maximize neuroplasticity and improve movement, memory, and cognition.

STEP ONE TO MAXIMIZE NEUROPLASTICITY:

EXTREME FOCUS!

Extreme focus or hyper focus is the first step in maximizing neuroplasticity.

You can CHOOSE to direct your focus. Here is an example.

If I ask you "how do your feet feel inside your shoes right now?" – chances are, you were not thinking about your feet until I asked you how they feel. Now that you have directed attention to your feet, you are choosing to focus on how your feet feel.

In the words of Stanford professor and neuroscientist, Dr. Andrew Huberman, this direction of attention is referred to as:

SELF DIRECTED ADAPTIVE NEUROPLASTICITY

And, if you have not already, be sure to check out Dr. Huberman's podcast. It is the most amazing and articulate neuroscience education I have ever come upon. Much of the information in this chapter is pulled from Huberman's research and education.

Let's go through the learning process and look at what happens and how you might *feel* while engaging in a learning event.

- You decide you want to learn to do something: a new skill or movement
- Every time you enter the practice of learning this new skill, we will call it a **learning event**
- Practice "chunking" (small blocks of time of hyper focus). This may be 30 seconds, one minute, 3 minutes, etc. where you HYPER FOCUS while doing the activity or skill you wish to develop
- Ignore all outside distractions to the best of your ability, HYPER FOCUS and practice the new skill or movement
- Do it until you feel "agitation" for a while (the amount of agitation time will vary depending on what you are practicing and how you feel doing it)
- Perhaps you are learning a new multitasking skill and after 30 seconds, you start to feel agitation or that you are exercising extreme effort (more-so mentally than physically in most cases)
- Push yourself (don't kill yourself) and feel this agitation for 15, 20, 30 seconds. Then, take a break and repeat

That feeling of strain during the effort is the release of **NORADRENALINE.**

- The release of noradrenaline may cause the *feeling* of strain and discomfort during effort

Additionally, during focused effort, **ACETYLCHOLINE** is released at the synapses involved of what is being learned

- **ACETYLCHOLINE** marks these neurons for strengthening
- The more you practice the new skill, the more the synapses occur between neurons and the more they become marked for the strengthening and the development of new neural pathways

(Andrew Huberman, 2020)

STEP TWO TO MAXIMIZE NEUROPLASTICITY:

SLEEP!

As we already mentioned, acetylcholine marks neurons for strengthening during focused effort.

This strengthening occurs during sleep or a sleep like state (Andrew Huberman, 2020).

It may take several nights or a week or more of sleep for neurons to firmly develop. Practicing your new skills daily is imperative to realize maximum results.

Eventually, after enough practice followed by enough sleep, you will one day wake up and perform the new skill with ease.

Your new neural firing pathways will have developed, and you will improve the skill you set out to learn or perform better.

What happens next? That is up to you, but my advice is, keep practicing the skills you develop, but make them more challenging and work towards getting proficient at the next level of performing the skill.

Many times, during focused activity, the feeling of strain can make us want to give up. I have three words to say about that: **DON'T GIVE UP!**

ATTACH A REWARD TO YOUR EFFORT

During the short bouts of focused effort, attach a reward to the event, for example: "this is me getting better" or "this is me reducing fall risk" or "this is me learning to move better."

Attaching reward will help to keep you focused and drive you towards achieving your goal.

Do you have trouble getting motivated to do your exercises? In the next chapter, we will talk about the many roles of dopamine and help you to get started!

CHAPTER SUMMARY:

1: Hyper focus during each learning event
2: Attach reward to the agitation you feel
3: SLEEP (learn how to optimize sleep in chapter 5)

Chapter 4

The Many Roles of Dopamine

Dopamine is an organic chemical (a neurotransmitter) of the catecholamine and phenethylamine families that plays several essential roles in the brain and body such as movement, pleasure, motivation, memory, or attention, among many others. (Unknown, 2019)

We know that in Parkinson's disease, production of dopamine is diminished, and movement (and often cognition and memory) are compromised.

Dopamine replacement medications can be helpful in raising dopamine activity in the brain but tend to have a short-term affect. This is the primary reason many people with PD take dopamine replacement medications 3-4 times per day. The increased dopamine activity helps to temporarily improve movement (and perhaps cognition and mental clarity).

When a medication is fully effective, we call this an "ON" period (where the person with PD moves and performs better). As the medication wears off, they will go into an "OFF" period where they are not moving and performing as well. Every person is uniquely affected by PD and will respond differently to dopamine replacement medications. In addition, effectiveness of medications may vary from day to day and higher dosages of these meds are usually needed as the disease progresses.

What is dopamine responsible for?

This subject goes deep, but I will break it down as simply as I can as dopamine has many roles and we will soon discover how a lack of dopamine can exacerbate PD symptoms and quality of life.

Dopamine plays a very important role in:

- Movement
- Coordination
- Balance
- Mental clarity
- Memory
- Cognition
- Motivation
- Goal seeking
- Behavior
- Sleep
- Attention
- Mood

For example – when we look at diminished dopamine in a person living with PD, it is common to see a lack of motivation. Dopamine is a "driver" towards goals and a lack of dopamine can cause overall diminished motivation.

I see it every single day. One of my many patients with Parkinson's will want to cancel a therapy session or they show up at my clinic and want to do as little as possible.

Caregivers often report the person with PD being a "couch potato."

Lack of motivation is common, but with encouragement and support, the person with PD can develop new habits that "get them off the couch and moving more."

Is there simple way to deal with this lack of motivation? From personal experience, I say YES! My advice is super simple: JUST GET STARTED and you will get the energy to keep doing what you set out to do.

But *simple* does not necessarily mean *easy.*

We will learn why in the following pages.

Let's look deeper into the roles of dopamine

Information in this section is primarily taken from my favorite book about dopamine entitled, **"The Molecule of More"** by David Z. Lieberman, MD and Michael E. Long. (Long, 2018)

- Dopamine needs something to do
- Dopamine is focused on the future

- Dopamine is designed to maximize future resources

Primal roles of dopamine (the good stuff)

- Dopamine is a driver towards survival (eating, reproduction, goals, etc.)
- Dopamine drives us towards achievement
  - An accomplishment (i.e., sales goal, completing a marathon, getting a degree, finding a mate, finishing writing a book, an exercise session, etc.)

Dopamine drives the "pursuit" of survival and feeling happy or accomplished.

Dopamine works to drive creativity (music, art, dance, writing, etc.)

Dopamine was designed to drive these actions. This is the good stuff.

The negative side of dopamine

Dopamine can have a negative side and lead to addictions or addictive tendencies. For example, when someone commits a crime and gets away with it, a huge dopamine rush will give the feeling of a sense of accomplishment.

When someone shoots heroin or snorts cocaine (or ingests any other addictive substances), there is a huge rush of dopamine which causes a feeling of elation.

Food, cigarettes, alcohol, and sugar can be highly addicting (along with potato chips and countless other foods that make you temporarily feel good). When we drink the drink, eat the cookie, eat the potato chip, snort the cocaine, etc. we get the feeling of satisfaction or being "high."

The first time we try these things, the dopamine rush is enormous, and the sense of elation is the best feeling! But what happens next? We want MORE. Hence the title of Lieberman's book, "The Molecule of More."

Addicts will pursue the feeling again and again, but seldom will the "high" feel the same as the first time. Dopamine drives us towards pursuing that initial feeling of elation and thus can easily lead to an addiction.

These are external sources of dopamine: food, sugar, alcohol, cigarettes, drugs, sex, another person, etc.

These behaviors and actions have ruined the lives of countless people. They have led to health problems, financial problems, marital problems, obesity, and death.

Creating dopamine from within

While levodopa and other dopamine replacement medications are necessary and very helpful for a person living with PD, we can take advantage of the brains ability to create its own dopamine from within. How do we do this?

In my clinic, I have beautiful gifts from people all over the world. Each gift was given to me by a person living with Parkinson's or some other type of movement disorder.

Even better, each gift was hand-made by the person who gave it to me!

I have paintings, drawings, pottery, and other gifts created by these wonderful friends.

Here's a game changer for you. They create these works of art because it makes them feel good while they're creating it.

Extra dopamine is produced and what's REALLY cool is that they're symptoms (tremors, dyskinesia, anxiety, etc.) diminish greatly during the creation of the piece of art.

For the person with PD, creating dopamine from within is one of the best ways of managing disease symptoms.

JUST GET STARTED

As stated by best-selling author and Harvard professor, Dr. John Ratey; "the human body is designed to move." Maybe you don't want to move (I feel that way often), but once you get moving, you'll feel different, and you'll want to keep moving.

Movement lights up the brain and fires up all kinds of synaptic firing activity. Movement also produces chemicals, hormones, and neurotransmitters (and lights up their pathways), including dopamine. Movement will give you energy.

So, JUST GET STARTED! It's that simple.

No matter what it is you want to do (or don't want to do but know you need to do), JUST GET STARTED.

Parkinson's and dopamine: Finding balance

There are SO many ways to fire up dopamine circuits from within. Find what you LIKE to do and do it!

Here are a few ideas that have helped people I know who live with PD:

- Exercise (find what you WILL do and then do it)
  - Bicycling
  - Weightlifting
  - Yoga
  - CrossFit
  - Running
  - Tennis
  - Badminton
  - Ping pong
  - Walking
  - Hiking
  - Swimming
  - Etc.
- Dance
- Group fitness
- Rock Steady Boxing
- Creating pottery
- Painting
- Drawing
- Socializing

Beware of creating too much dopamine

Parkinson's is a complicated disease and each person with PD is uniquely affected differently and yes, it is possible to create too much dopamine.

How do we know if too much dopamine is being produced?

Typical indications may include:

- Sudden urge to gamble
- The urge to shop far more than usual
- Hypersexuality
- Unusual binge-like behaviors

While this doesn't happen often, it is possible that when a person with PD begins an exercise program, the increased dopamine created during exercise may create the need for a lower dose of dopamine replacement medications.

Don't let this prevent you from starting an exercise program. For most people with Parkinson's, an exercise program is VERY much needed and as described in my first book, engaging in exercise can help to slow disease progression and manage disease symptoms.

However, if you find yourself wanting to engage in unusual behaviors, call your neurologist right away, explain what you are feeling, and follow their recommendations.

Chapter Summary

- Dopamine is diminished in production in PD

- Exercise is necessary and gets blood and oxygen to the brain, creates BDNF, fires up dopamine activity, and helps slow disease progression.
- Dopamine replacement medications will help to improve movement, cognition, and performance
- Creating dopamine from within is highly beneficial in managing disease symptoms
- Find healthy activities and exercises you like to do and do them
- JUST GET STARTED and you'll get the energy to keep going

Understanding the roles of dopamine and how to create it will help you towards improving your movement and quality of life.

Chapter 5

Manage Sleep Effectively

People with Parkinson's often times experience problems with sleep (and so do many other people).

This short chapter will teach you how to set up your sleep cycle upon waking in the morning. Starting your day like this will help you to get to sleep better and stay asleep for longer.

This information applies to all people (except those who are completely blind). Additionally, the education in this chapter comes from two sources:

- A book entitled "Why We Sleep: Unlocking the Power of Sleep and Dreams" by Dr. Matthew Walker (Walker, 2017)
- Huberman Podcast: Dr. Andrew Huberman (Huberman, 2021)

Why We Sleep

Sleep enriches a diversity of functions within the brain, including our ability to learn, memorize, and make logical decisions and choices. Sleep recalibrates our emotional brain circuits, allowing us to navigate next-day social and psychological challenges with cool-headed composure (Walker, 2017)

In the body, sleep builds up our immune system, helping to prevent infection and ward off sickness. Sleep reforms the body's metabolic state by fine-tuning the balance of insulin and circulating glucose. (Walker, 2017)

Sleep also helps to regulate our appetite, helping to control body weight through healthy food selection rather than rash impulsivity. Sufficient sleep maintains a flourishing microbiome within your gut from which we know so much of our nutritional health begins. Adequate sleep is intimately tied to the fitness of our cardiovascular system, lowering blood pressure while helping keep our hearts in fine condition. (Walker, 2017)

Needless to say, we need our sleep as it will help with overall physical, mental, and emotional well-being and help us to live a longer and healthier life.

The information in this section applies to those who are waking up during daylight hours or just before sunrise and going to bed when it is dark outside or just prior to total darkness. If you are doing shiftwork, please refer to www.thepdbook.org for protocol.

Setting up your sleep-wake cycle

Step 1: Upon Waking

- first thing in the morning, expose your eyes to natural light for a couple of minutes or more
  - ideally, this means that you go outside and look up! Look towards the sky (but don't look directly into the sun)
  - looking through a window is better than not taking in natural light, but being outside will help to set up your sleep-wake cycle better than looking through a window
  - it doesn't matter if it is cloudy or sunny. You want to take in natural daylight from above

The cells in the lower part of the retina are constantly viewing what is above us. When these cells sense light after sleeping, the activation of the sleep-wake cycle should begin.

How and why does this occur?

The eyes are a part of the brain, and the retina has cells that are designed to detect sunlight. These cells primarily reside in the lower half of the retina. (Huberman, 2021)

Because of the location of these cells in the retina, they are continually sensing light (or lack of light) from above. They are viewing our upper visual field. (Huberman, 2021)

Once these cells detect light from above, they trigger the brain into kicking in the wake cycle. This creates the production of cortisol and starts an internal clock within your body and brain setting you up to stay awake for approximately 14-17 hours (this number varies from person to person). (Huberman, 2021)

As you go through your day, your sleep-wake cycle clock is ticking.

Eventually, it will be time to go to sleep at night.

Step 2: Setting up the sleep cycle

- an hour or so prior to sundown, step outside and look up at the sky for a couple of minutes (avoid looking at direct sunlight)
  - again, it is best to be outside and look up rather than looking through a window
  - it doesn't matter if it is cloudy or sunny. You want to take in natural daylight from above

Viewing natural light from above before sundown triggers the brain to produce melatonin, a hormone that helps us get to sleep.

This simple sleep-wake cycle process can be a game changer for those who have difficulty sleeping.

Other important considerations

After going to sleep at night, it is important to avoid bright light.

For example, perhaps you need to use the bathroom. If you feel safe walking in the dark (and have the ability to navigate to the bathroom without tripping or falling), walk in the dark or place a very dim light lower on your horizon (i.e., nightlight in an outlet near the floor).

Especially between the hours of approximately 11:00pm and 4:00am, it is important to avoid bright light, if possible. (Huberman, 2021)

Exposure to bright light from above during these hours are likely to trigger your wake cycle, causing difficulty getting back to sleep. (Huberman, 2021)

Turning on an overhead hallway, bedroom, or bathroom light may trigger the wake cycle prematurely.

Looking at your phone, tablet, or computer may prematurely trigger the wake cycle.

Do your best to practice the process outlined above. This may be the answer to better sleep for you!

Chapter 6

The Importance of Nutrition in Parkinson's Disease

Written by: MCSP Cynthia Karyna López-Botello

Introduction

Nutrition science talks about the nature and distribution of nutrients in food, how these nutrients affect the metabolism of living beings, and the possible consequences that can be caused by insufficient or excessive food intake. For this reason, nutrition is essential during all stages of life to maintain good health. In neurological diseases, nutrition is compromised, causing serious consequences. Such is the case of Parkinson's Disease, which is associated with nutritional problems such as malnutrition caused by involuntary weight loss, loss of muscle mass and gastrointestinal problems such as constipation. Adequate nutritional treatment as part of transdisciplinary care is essential so that people with Parkinson's disease can lead a good quality of life.

Nutritional Status

Nutritional status is understood as the balance that exists between energy intake and energy expenditure. The energy intake comes from the consumption of foods with a good nutritional value and the energy expenditure is the relationship that exists between the consumption of energy from food and the energy that the body uses to correctly perform its functions. To obtain balance and obtain good nutritional status, the energy consumed must be equal to that expended by the body.

In most Parkinson's cases, there is no adequate balance in nutritional status. At one extreme, there are those patients with a higher energy expenditure caused by involuntary movements, thus causing a noticeable weight loss, which in severe cases leads to malnutrition and loss of muscle mass. On the other hand, there are those patients who have an excessive food intake, with little energy expenditure, causing problems with overweight and obesity (these cases are scarcer, and it is more common to find weight loss in patients).

There are several factors that favor weight loss in Parkinson's disease, among which include gastrointestinal disorders such as constipation, loss of appetite, difficulty passing or swallowing food (also known as dysphagia) and as mentioned previously – increased energy expenditure arising from symptoms of stiffness, tremor, and dyskinesias. Weight loss has been associated with a poor quality of life in patients and a rapid progression of the disease. Therefore, the role of the nutritionist throughout the Parkinson's disease stages is essential to prevent serious consequences from happening and to help the patient lead a better quality of life.

To maintain a good nutritional state during the illness, it is important to have a balanced diet that is adequate to the personal needs of each patient. There has been a lot of controversy on the issue of proper diet in Parkinson's patients, however, one of the most important aspects to consider is to stop involuntary weight loss and increase muscle mass.

Parkinson's Disease Diet

To determine the type of diet that a Parkinson's patient should follow, it is important to first know the role that each nutrient play in the body during illness and the interaction that can exist between medications and nutrients from foods.

Energy Intake

Due to the malnutrition present in most cases of Parkinson's, it is important to emphasize the importance of necessary energy intake during this pathology. As we have previously mentioned, each patient is different and each one will have a different nutritional status, as well as different symptoms of the disease. Due to characteristic symptoms of the disease such as tremor and stiffness, a greater number of calories must be provided per day to avoid the excess energy expenditure that can lead to weight loss. Hypercaloric eating plans are normally recommended to counteract involuntary weight loss.

Fats or Lipids

There are several types of fats that are considered essential for the proper functioning of the body. Among the most important essential fats during the treatment of Parkinson's Disease is Omega 3. It has been proven in several studies that a supplementation of this fat helps to increase the levels of dopamine in the brain and decrease neuroinflammation. This happens by their anti-inflammatory properties. In addition to finding these Omega 3's in the presentation of supplements, there are several foods that have them such as tuna, salmon, soybean oil, flaxseed, canola oil and in certain nuts such as almonds, walnuts, peanuts, and others.

Proteins and their Interaction with Levodopa

Proteins are one of the primary and most important nutrients for treating Parkinson's disease. Studies have already shown that muscle mass of both female and male patients is severely affected by unintentional weight loss. Therefore, protein is a nutrient that cannot be left out and diets must supply enough protein to avoid serious consequences. However, an important factor to consider is that proteins of animal origin such as dairy, cheese, meat, fish, chicken, and eggs, create an interaction with one of the most essential medications for the treatment of disease, which is levodopa, specifically at the level of brain receptors.

For this reason, special care must be taken in the diet prescribed to patients. The nutritional objective is that both the protein and the medicine are correctly absorbed by the body and thus prevent the progression of the disease. Various investigations carried out worldwide have created experiments with different types of diets, some where there is a low proportion of animal protein, another where protein redistribution is made, and another that adjusts food consumption together with the drug to avoid competing in absorption. Offering patients a diet with a low proportion of protein of animal origin carries the risk of consequences. This happens because we can put the patient's muscle mass at risk and cause sarcopenia, which is defined as muscle malnutrition. Parkinson's disease affects all patients differently, therefore, it is very important to assess the nutritional status of each patient to determine the indicated diet according to their needs.

Not all patients have this high sensitivity to dietary proteins, therefore, it is important to be evaluated by a nutrition professional in order to prepare an individualized eating plan. In my professional experience as a nutritionist specializing in Parkinson's disease, one of the diets that have worked best with patients is the one where it is decided to redistribute the proteins during the day. Proteins of animal origin are distributed in the evening to avoid a bad absorption of the drug, however, it is important that dinner is not consumed too late in the evening, because intestinal mobility is reduced and can cause gastrointestinal disorders. During the day, patients consume a higher proportion of vegetable proteins, which can be found in beans, lentils, chickpeas, among others.

Another highly recommended diet alternative is one with an amount of protein balanced according to the weight of the patient, normally according to the needs of each person, 1.5 to 2 grams / kilogram of the patient's healthy weight is recommended. The amount reached is divided into the main mealtimes in equal amounts. This meal plan will offer the required amount of protein individually and thus be somewhat reduced compared to other methods. An important fact is that the levodopa medication must be consumed from 30 minutes to 1 hour before each meal.

Vitamins and Minerals

The consumption of vitamins is essential for the proper functioning of the body. In recent years, vitamins have become more important in Parkinson's disease. B vitamins play an important role as enzyme cofactors helping to regulate metabolism, improving the function of the nervous system, and promoting growth and cell division. Among all the B vitamins, only those that perform the most important functions in Parkinson's disease will be mentioned.

Vitamin B3 or also known as Niacin, is responsible for eliminating all toxic chemicals from the body, in addition, it participates in the production of steroid hormones. This vitamin is found in various foods such as coffee, meat, eggs, wheat, tomatoes, among others. Furthermore, it can also be synthesized from tryptophan. A deficiency of this vitamin can cause dermatitis, diarrhea and in some cases depression and in one study it was suggested that an excess of it was related to the evolution of Parkinson's disease. The consumption of this vitamin in low doses helps neuroprotection and works as an antioxidant, but when its intake is not controlled it can lead to neurotoxicity, specifically dopaminergic.

Likewise, a possible interaction between the medications of Sinemet or Madopar with vitamin B3 has been found. This happens because carbidopa or benserazide can inhibit the synthesis of the vitamin, therefore, it is important to have a diet with foods that provide an adequate amount of this vitamin.

Vitamin B6 or pyridoxine, is also part of the B complex. This vitamin has the function of intervening in the brain substances that are in charge of regulating mood, as is the case of serotonin. Therefore, it is important to administer sufficient amounts, especially in those patients with sleep disturbances, depression, and stress. Foods with a good content of vitamin B6 include salmon, tuna, whole grains, legumes, broccoli, peppers, avocado, among others.

Antioxidants also play an important role during Parkinson's disease. Among the most essential is, vitamin C, also called ascorbic acid. It is responsible for significantly reducing oxidative stress and is involved in many other functions such as collagen synthesis, carnitine synthesis, cholesterol metabolism, amino acid absorption, and regulation of some hormones. In the metabolism of dopamine, oxidative stress occurs, which causes an accumulation of abnormal proteins in Parkinson's disease. Therefore, an adequate consumption of ascorbic acid can protect the patient from toxicity by levodopa and also increase the absorption of the drug. Vitamin C is essential in brain development. We can find it in the following foods: orange, lemon, grapefruit, mandarin, kiwi, spinach, strawberries, raspberries, blackberries, peppers, among others.

Vitamin E is also a powerful antioxidant that participates in cognitive, immune, physical performance and also protects the body's tissues from substances called free radicals. In Parkinson's disease, several researchers have shown that a high consumption of this vitamin can help prevent the disease from occurring and prolong treatment with levodopa. There is still insufficient evidence to prove this function well, but its antioxidant function can help protect against oxidative stress. Some foods with high content of vitamin E, are, olive oil, asparagus, chard, mango, among others.

Lastly, vitamin D is considered a steroid hormone that aids in calcium absorption and bone health. This vitamin is related to Parkinson's disease because it protects dopaminergic neurons from neurotoxicity. Many studies have shown that adequate supplementation of this vitamin can attenuate the deterioration of Parkinson's disease and decrease the risk of fractures in patients. Among the foods with the highest content of this vitamin are: salmon, sardines, and tuna – but vitamin D is especially obtained from the sun.

Finally, to conclude with the most important nutrients we will talk about minerals. Like vitamins, some minerals play an essential role in slowing the progression of Parkinson's Disease and an adequate consumption of these minerals either through the diet or supplemented is necessary. Among the most important functions of minerals are, the formation of bones, production of new hormones, and improved functioning of the heart. Here are some of the most important ones.

An accumulation of iron has often been found in the brain in patients with Parkinson's disease, especially in the substantia nigra and the basal ganglia. This observed accumulation may be due to a dysfunction of iron homeostasis in the brain. Several studies have verified that a high consumption of this mineral is related to an increased risk of Parkinson's disease, however, it is a mineral that also performs important functions such as the formation of blood cells in the body. For this reason, iron intake should be adjusted to the needs of each patient to avoid the risk of consuming excess. Among the foods with the highest content are nuts, whole grains, legumes, among others.

Magnesium is a mineral that helps protect neurons. A deficiency can increase the damage caused by toxic substances. It is very easy to obtain through the diet since it is mainly found in nuts, tuna, and green vegetables. Due to its regulating and toning function of the muscles, it may help Parkinson's disease patients who have symptoms of muscle stiffness, however, there is still little evidence about this relationship.

Constipation

More than 50% of Parkinson's disease patients suffer constipation. It is one of the most common symptoms and may even have an impact on the patient's emotional and psychological state. Several studies have shown that proper supplementation of dietary fiber and probiotics can help improve it. The modification of the patient's lifestyle, thus increasing the consumption of fiber from fruits, vegetables, and whole grains, together with an adequate consumption of natural water, helps significantly to decrease it, since it increases intestinal motility.

It is important to mention that the consumption of fruits and vegetables should be together with the peel, since when removing it, the amount of fiber decreases considerably. In patients who have difficulty passing food, it is recommended to cook food slightly to avoid choking.

Conclusion

Even though nutrition has not been proven to cure the disease, good nutrition as prescribed by a qualified professional may help to slow disease progression. It is important that all appropriate changes are made together with a nutrition professional so as not to alter other functions of the organism. A healthy diet very much helps to improve the quality of life of patients with Parkinson's disease.

References

Avallone, R., Vitale, G., & Bertolotti, M. (2019). Omega-3 Fatty Acids and Neurodegenerative Diseases: New Evidence in Clinical Trials. *International Journal of Molecular Sciences, 20*(4256), 1-22.

Barichella, M., Cereda, E., Cassani, E., Pinelli, G., Iorio, L., Ferri, V., . . . Pezzoli, G. (2017). Dietary habits and neurological features of Parkinson's disease patients: Implications for practice. *Clinical Nutrition, 36*(4), 1054-1061.

Ciulla, M., Marinelli, L., Cacciatore, I., & Di Stefano, A. (2019). Role of Dietary Supplements in the Management of. *Biomolecules, 9*(271), 1-23.

Li, P., & Song, C. (2020). Potential treatment of Parkinson's disease with omega-3 polyunsaturated fatty acids. *International Journal on Nutrition, Diet and Nervous System*, 1-13.

López-Botello, C., González-Peña, S., Berrún-Castañón, L., Estrada-Bellmann, I., & Ancer-Rodríguez, P. (2017). Nutritional Status in patients with Parkinson's Disease at a third-level hospital in Northeastern México. *Medicina Universitaria, 19*(75), 45-49.

Ma, K., Xiong, N., Shen, Y., Han, C., Liu, L., Zhang, G., . . . Wang, T. (2018). Weight Loss and Malnutrition in

Patients with Parkinson's Disease: Current Knowledge and Future Prospects. *Aging Neuroscience, 10*(1), 1-10.

Pedrosa, A., Timmermann, L., & Pedrosa, D. (2018). Management of constipation in patients with Parkinson's. *Nature Partners Journals, 6,* 1-10.

Rodríguez, M., Villar, A., Valencia, C., & Cervantes, A. (2011). Características epidemiológicas de pacientes con enfermedad de Parkinson de un hospital de referencia en México. *Neurociencia, 16*(2), 64-68.

Seidi, S., Santiago, J., Bilyk, H., & Potashkin, J. (2014). The emerging role of nutrition in Parkinson's disease. *Front Aging Neurosci., 6*(36), 1-14.

Sherzai, A., Tagliati, M., Park, K., Pezeshkian, S., & Sherzai, D. (2016). Micronutrients and Risk of Parkinson's Disease: A Systematic Review. *Gerontology & Geriatric Medicine, 2,* 1-12.

Virmani, T., Tazan, S., Mazzoni, P., Ford, B., & Greene, P. (2016). Motor fluctuations due to interaction between dietary protein and levodopa in Parkinson's disease. *Journal of Clinical Movement Disorders, 3*(8), 1-7.

Wang, A., Lin, Y., Wu, Y., & Zhang, D. (2015). Macronutrients intake and risk of Parkinson's disease: A meta-analysis. *Geriatr Gerontol Int, 15*(5), 606-616.

Zhao, X., Zhang, M., Li, C., Jiang, X., Su, Y., & Zhang, Y. (2019). Benefits of Vitamins in the Treatment of

Parkinson's Disease. *Oxidative Medicine and Cellular Longevity*, 1-14.

Chapter 7

Benefits of Using Power Plate® and Vibration Therapy

As discussed in my first book, vibration therapy has proven to be highly effective in reducing Parkinson's symptoms and improving movement, and has a multitude of additional benefits, as well.

The implementation of vibration therapy prior to a workout or activity generally leads to a better movement or exercise experience. Try using the appropriate vibration techniques BEFORE exercising. This will help to wake up the central nervous system, peripheral nervous system, and brain.

While there are a multitude of companies providing vibration products, I exclusively use Power Plate® products for any form of vibration therapy. They make a variety of vibration devices. and the quality of their products are unparalleled.

Whole Body Vibration

Whole body vibration (WBV) has shown to be an effective technique to help improve balance, stability, and gait in people with PD. The Power Plate® has benefitted a wide variety of populations.

Whole body vibration on the Power Plate® works like this; after stepping onto the Power Plate® platform, you set the machine to create a consistent, controlled level of vibration. This is referred to as a harmonic wave as the platform moves up and down, forward, and back, and side to side.

You will feel a destabilizing effect on your body and as the device moves, your muscles will react to stabilize your body. The platform produces 25 to 50 vibrations per second, at precisely controlled amplitudes, which triggers reflexive muscular contractions. (Powell, 2014)

Although it may feel strange at first, you quickly get used to the sensation! People with PD almost always feel a sense of being "connected" once again. They feel positive effects and this transfers to activities of daily living including balance, stability, and gait.

Clinical research indicates that whole body vibration improves gait performance in people with Parkinson's disease (Silvia Marazzi, 2020) in addition to beneficial effects on balance, stability, and mobility in individuals with Parkinson disease (Sharareh Sharififar, 2014).

The benefits of Power Plate® have been recognized by the medical profession and studies have shown an abundance of health benefits can be gained including (Powell, 2014):

1. Improved muscle strength and power
2. Improved flexibility and range of motion
3. Reduced pain and soreness with faster recovery

4. Increased bone mineral density and prevention of bone mineral density loss related to ageing
5. Improved circulation, cardiovascular and cardiorespiratory functions
6. Improved balance, mobility, and strength among the elderly and inactive population (Powell, 2014)

Segmental Vibration Tools

In my clinic, we use the Power Plate® WBV platform many times during every session and execute countless exercises that would normally be done of the floor, for example: squats, bicep curls, lateral raises, single leg strength and balance exercises and much more.

For a video library of exercises using the Power Plate® WBV platform, visit the book support website at: www.thepdbook.org

We also do a lot with other **Power Plate®** vibration tools in the way of segmental vibration therapy. Let's take a look.

Power Plate® DualSphere is perfect for effective, concentrated massage. Featuring a unique contoured shape and exclusive textured design, the DualSphere is ideal for targeting hard to reach areas including feet, neck and back to help relax and rejuvenate tight and sore

muscles, release fascia and promote blood flow to help you prepare faster and recover quicker.

The DualSphere is a cutting-edge vibrating massager that:

- Helps relax and rejuvenate tight and sore muscles
- Enhances range of motion

- Promotes blood flow and fascia release

- Reduces pain

- Accelerates exercise warm up and recovery (Plate, Power Plate, n.d.)

Power Plate® Pulse is a best-in-class premium, powerful, yet whisper quiet, portable handheld massager. It helps relax and rejuvenate tight and sore muscles, release fascia and promote blood flow to help you prepare faster and recover quicker. With more attachments than any other massager on the market, you can choose between six different options suited for various warm-up and recovery needs.

Includes a travel case.

The Pulse is a cutting-edge vibrating massager that:

- Helps relax and rejuvenate tight and sore muscles

- Enhances range of motion

- Promotes blood flow and fascia release (Plate, Power Plate, n.d.)

The Power Plate® Mini+ ™ is an ultracompact, quiet, portable handheld massager that gives you a relaxing, reenergizing massage wherever your day takes you. Conveniently sized to fit into a purse, backpack, or sports bag, the Power Plate Mini+ can give you quality treatment, anytime, anywhere.

The Mini+™ is an extremely versatile, lightweight massager that:

- Relaxes and rejuvenates tight and sore muscles

- Accelerates exercise warm up and recovery

- Promotes blood flow and fascia release

- Enhances range of motion and reduces muscle pain

What's Included

The Power Plate Mini+ comes with two unique attachments to suit your preparation and recovery as well as the USB-C charging cable and a lightweight carrying pouch for storage and travel. (Plate, Power Plate, n.d.)

Power Plate® Roller™ takes classic foam rolling to a new level, the Power Plate Roller is a portable vibrating massager that helps relax and rejuvenate tight and sore muscles, release fascia and promote blood flow to help you prepare faster and recover quicker.

The Roller is a cutting-edge vibrating massager that:

- Helps relax and rejuvenate tight and sore muscles

- Enhances range of motion

- Promotes blood flow and fascia release (Plate, Power Plate, n.d.)

Choosing the best vibration tool to use

This will depend on what body part you are looking to massage.

If another person is administering the massage, it will be up to you and the person administering to choose the best device (and attachment).

If doing a self-massage, it can be difficult to use a hand-held device to access certain areas, i.e.: upper traps, back, glutes, and other areas. For these hard-to-reach areas, when self-massaging, choose a device such as the DualSphere or Roller.

Additional advice

When striving for fascia release, vibrating devices are to be used on muscles, not bones. Bones don't change shape!

Additionally, remember these three things; if it numbs, tingles or pulses, STOP! Numbing and tingling means you are likely on a nerve. Pulsing indicates you are likely on a blood supply.

Segmental Vibration Areas:

Plantar skin stimulation

Stimulating the plantar skin has countless benefits that help to improve balance, reaction time, and movement.

This can be done on the Power Plate® WBV platform. We also find the DualSphere or Roller to be highly effective for stimulating plantar skin nerves which greatly increases sensory input to the brain which will help to improve movement.

Application: Ideally, it is best to place the DualSphere or Roller on the floor on a carpeted or soft surface (e.g., a pillow or folded up yoga mat) and not a hard surface such as tile or wood. Turn it on, have a seat in the chair, and place your foot (barefoot, no socks) on the device.

We recommend using a low-speed setting first and increase vibration speed as you see fit. Very slowly, move your foot around on the device and cover as much plantar skin area as possible. Continue moving your foot for at least a couple of minutes or longer, if possible. Repeat on the other foot.

Tremors / Palmar skin stimulation

Often times, people with PD experience the resting tremor of a limb or limbs. Stimulation of the palm skin not only helps to wake up the central nervous system, peripheral nervous system, and brain, but can help to temporarily reduce tremors.

Application: Turn on the DualSphere and hold it in your hands. Be sure the device is in contact with as much palm and finger skin as possible. Hold the device firmly for 5-10 minutes or until you feel you have had enough vibration. Turn off and set down the device and observe the tremors. Is there a difference? It is likely they are significantly diminished or gone.

While the diminished tremors will be temporary (usually between a few minutes to a couple of hours), it can be very helpful when the person with PD is preparing to do anything requiring fine motor skills: texting, writing, typing, buttoning a button, zipping a zipper, brushing teeth, using an eating utensil, etc.

I know many people with PD who stopped going out to dinner because they are self-conscious about their tremors and are concerned that they will spill food or a drink. But there's good news! Purchase a DualSphere and hold it during the trip to the restaurant while someone else drives. Upon arrival, their tremors are nearly always diminished to a point (or gone completely) where they can eat and drink without worrying about spilling anything. This can be highly beneficial in boosting confidence and self-esteem.

Restless Legs Syndrome (RLS)

Straight from the Mayo Clinic database: "Restless legs syndrome (RLS) is a condition that causes an uncontrollable urge to move your legs, usually because of an uncomfortable sensation. It typically happens in the evening or nighttime hours when you are sitting or lying down. Moving temporarily eases the unpleasant feeling.

Restless legs syndrome, also known as Willis-Ekbom disease, can begin at any age and generally worsens as you age. It can disrupt sleep, which interferes with daily activities." (Clinic M. , Restless legs syndrome, n.d.)

It is common for people with PD to experience RLS, sometimes many years before diagnosis. Vibration can help significantly reduce RLS.

Application: Prior to sleeping, position yourself on a bed or couch with legs in front of you. Choose a leg, take the vibrating device, and very slowly move it over the muscles. While there is no specific pattern you need to follow, perhaps start on your quadricep. Next, place the device under your leg and work on the hamstrings. Then, place it under the calve and slowly cover as much area as possible. Repeat on the other leg.

Moving the device SLOWLY is the key. I highly recommend spending a minimum of 5 minutes on each leg. The more time spent, the more benefits will be realized.

Dystonia

Various types of dystonia are common in the Parkinson's population. A few examples include foot, cervical, and abdominal dystonia, in additional to generalized dystonia. Dystonia can be idiopathic, genetic, or acquired.

Dystonia is an involuntary contraction of muscles and can vary from mild to severe. A miscommunication between nerve cells in the basal ganglia (the area of the brain responsible for inhibiting muscle contractions) can cause dystonia in one or more areas of the body.

The involuntary muscle contractions cause repetitive clenching and/or twisting movements which can cause pain, cramping, and less than optimal posture.

Foot dystonia: In our experience, this is the most common type of focal dystonia. This involves the involuntary contractions of the abductor hallucis and other muscles in the foot that draw the ball of the foot closer to the heel and many times causing plantar flexed and inverted foot position. This can last anywhere from a few minutes to a few days and maybe extremely painful.

Application: Just as we do when stimulating the plantar skin, it is best to place the vibrating device on the floor on a carpeted or soft surface (e.g., a pillow or folded up yoga mat) and not a hard surface such as tile or wood. Turn it on, have a seat on a couch or chair, and place your foot (barefoot, no socks) on the device. We recommend using a low-speed setting first and increase vibration speed as you see fit. Very slowly, move your foot around on the device, concentrating on areas where you feel the most discomfort. Continue moving your foot for as long as you can tolerate or until the clenching diminishes or goes away. Repeat on the other foot, if needed.

Cervical dystonia: The involuntary and painful contractions of neck muscles pull the head to one side and may cause an uncontrollable forward or backward tilt of the head. Medical treatment may include Botox type injections into contracted muscles. However, vibration has shown to be helpful in realizing a temporary and partial reduction of involuntary contractions and diminished pain.

Application: It is best to have another person assist with this therapy as it is difficult to self-administer (although you will find a self-administer technique on the support website). Have the client or patient sit in a chair. The assistant will stand behind the chair.

On a low-speed setting, place the Power Plate® Pulse or Power Plate® Mini+ ™ on the side where contractions are occurring. Very slowly move the device around the area of contracted muscles. Be careful not to come in contact with boney areas. Bones do not contract or relax and vibrating on a bone or on the skull will be painful and needs to be avoided. ONLY use the device on muscles.

It is doubtful that the head will return to a normal position. Your goal is to use vibration to temporarily relax the muscles. This, in turn will hopefully lead to a reduction in discomfort or pain.

The cervical dystonia video on the support website shows the process of vibrating contracted muscles; In addition, it shows a taping technique to help stimulate a contraction of muscles on the other side of the neck.

The combination of vibration and taping the opposite side has proven to be greatly beneficial for many people.

Abdominal dystonia: This involves an involuntary contraction of muscles in the abdomen and can be very painful.

Application: As with all vibration techniques for dystonia, you will get the best results by moving the vibrating device very slowly. On a bed or couch, lay on your back and place the device on your abdomen. Slowly roll over the muscles that are involuntarily contracting. Do this for as long as needed or as long as you can tolerate.

Generalized dystonia: This is a tough one, folks as it affects multiple muscle groups in the body.

Generalized dystonia can be very painful and debilitating, although whole body vibration and segmental vibration has proven to be somewhat helpful. People living with generalized dystonia are often times unable to coordinate self-administered therapy, depending on how they are affected. Help from another person may be necessary.

As with all vibration techniques for dystonia, you will get the best results by moving the chosen vibration device very slowly on any and all affected muscle groups. Use the device on each affected area for as long as you can tolerate. Even a temporary diminishment of involuntary contractions can lead to a temporary relief of some amount of pain.

Constipation

People with PD often times live with constipation. Vibration therapy can be helpful in relieving constipation.

Application: Seated in a comfortable chair or lying on your back on a bed or couch, start by placing the chosen vibrating device on your descending colon (just below left side of rib cage and down to the left side of the navel). On low speed (at first), slowly move the device over this area for 3-5 minutes (or longer, if tolerable). Next, move to the ascending colon (just below right side of rib cage and down to the right side of the navel). On low speed (at first), slowly move the device over this area for 3-5 minutes (or longer, if tolerable).

Wait a little while and see how you feel. If you don't make a trip to the bathroom, repeat the process throughout the day. If you haven't made a trip to the bathroom by the next morning, repeat the process throughout the day.

There is a good chance you will loosen things up and make a trip (or trips) to the bathroom on the first day. Our clients and workshop attendees have had tremendous results with this, and many make a trip within only a few minutes.

Menstrual cramps

Many women experience the discomfort of menstrual cramps. This vibration technique is for all women in childbearing years, not just women with PD. And, while Parkinson's effects twice as many men as women and is generally an age-related disease, there are many women living with PD who are still in the childbearing years and experiencing a monthly menstrual period.

Application: On a bed or couch, lay on your back and place the device on your abdomen. Slowly move the device over the areas of discomfort. Do this for as long as you wish. We know of countless women who use the device for an hour or more. Vibration has been highly effective in relieving menstrual cramps.

Myofascial release

Self-administered myofascial release (SMR) is an effective method for releasing tight muscles, reducing rigidity, and improving flexibility, range of motion around joints, and posture.

While SMR is remarkably effective, it is much more efficiently taught via video demonstrations. Go to the support website and visit the SMR tab on the menu. There, you will find an extensive video library broken down to specific muscles and how best to release them.

Be SURE to watch the *SMR Intro* video for especially important *safety points* prior to administering any SMR.

For more information on **Power Plate®**, visit the book support website at www.thepdbook.org and visit www.powerplate.com

Chapter 8

Improving Cognition, Memory, and Movement

My primary goal in this chapter is to succinctly deliver concepts, strategies, and exercises to improve:

- Movement

- Memory

- Cognition

- Reaction time

- Multitasking abilities

With the exception of multitasking exercises, we can work on the other areas independently.

In this chapter, you will find lists of exercises for each category: movement, cognition, memory, and reactive training.

Later in the chapter, we will discuss the idea of pulling exercises from two or more of these lists and using them simultaneously to improve multitasking abilities.

Why do this? Because it helps us to move better and reduce the risk of falling.

Safety

Before we begin, please remember that safety is of paramount importance.

Challenge your client but be mindful of their safety.

My first book has an entire set of chapters devoted to assessments. These assessments allow you to determine a client's risk of falling.

The Fun and Creativity Factor

The type of training we do offers seemingly endless opportunities to be creative and have fun during the process.

I'll take you through a similar process of how we work with clients and patients at my clinic but remember:

- Know your patient and their abilities
- Find out their biggest challenges with movement, memory, cognition
- Know their goals
- Design a program that includes exercises to help them reach their goals
- Get feedback when trying something new and know if they like the exercise or not
- Be creative and keep your patient engaged
- Have FUN!

Where to Begin

This will depend on your client, their goals, how they feel, and perhaps many other factors.

Improving movement is always a goal for our clients (gait, rotations, etc.). In light of this, in the beginning of our program, we generally start with some type of movement.

BUT FIRST (before we begin any movement-based exercises), we like to start immediately with some cognition / memory exercises. They can be super simple, for example:

- Deliver three words that you'll ask them to remember for the duration of the sessions
  - i.e.: green, cucumber, pickle
  - Who is the president of the USA?
  - Who is the vice president?
    - (Don't be surprised if your patient has to think a while to give you the correct answer or perhaps names a former president)

Do you get the idea? Ask simple questions and give them something to remember during your session. Frequently stop during the session and ask them to recite the words you gave them.

If three words are too easy, add three more. For example:

- Yellow, corn, banana

Notice that I have chosen a theme. Cucumbers are green and pickles are made from cucumbers (and are usually green).

Corn and bananas are usually yellow, etc.

Now, start your movement exercises.

We choose exercises via results of movement assessments in conjunction with the client's goals.

Many clients complain of weakness. This often contributes to their balance and movement challenges.

We can't have optimal balance without sufficient strength. In light of this, we will often choose strength- based exercises as our movements, for example:

- Sit-to-stands
- Squats
- Step-ups
- Step-up to balance
- Single leg squats
- Deadlifts
- Single leg deadlifts
- and in addition, a multitude of core, back, and upper body strength exercises

Some days, we will begin with other movement exercises, but in every session, we will always do a few exercises (to the client's level of ability) from this partial list:

- walking
- walking through an agility ladder
- walking through an agility ladder stepping every other rung (BIG steps)
- moving sideways (adding cross-feet patterns and perhaps through an agility ladder)
- walking on a treadmill
- walking on a treadmill sideways (adding cross-feet patterns)
- walking backwards
- walking backwards on a treadmill
- moving forward, sideways, and backwards over hurdles (our hurdles are 5.5" high)
- jumping through an agility ladder (forwards, sideways, and backwards)
- single leg jumping through an agility ladder (straight down the ladder forward, sideways, and backwards – adding in a zig-zag pattern in each direction, too)

- multi-directional jumping in a tic-tac-toe box (emulating the Shark Skill Test, but getting creative)
- boxing (heavy bag, speed bag, one-on-one with another person, safely of course)
- practicing rotations

The above list is just a fraction of movement exercises we work on.

Multitasking: combining movement with cognition / memory / hand-eye coordination exercises

In the interest of improving multitasking abilities, we can now start what I refer to as *STACKING.* Stacking involves a combination of an exercise from the list of movement exercises above (or any movement exercise you choose) with one or more exercise from any of the remaining lists in this chapter.

IMPORTANT NOTE: DURING ALL EXERCISES, REMEMBER TO MAXIMIZE NEUROPLASTICITY VIA THE TWO STEP PROCESS:

- HYPERFOCUS
- SLEEP
- REPEAT

THIS IS HOW A PERSON BEST DEVELOPS AND IMPROVES THE ABILITY TO PERFORM EVERY

TYPE OF MOVEMENT AND IMPROVE COGNITION, MEMORY, AND MULTITASKING ABILITIES.

DOMAINS OF COGNITION

Some of these are borrowed from my first book, Parkinson's Regeneration Training and they fit perfectly into this chapter to help tie things together. Let's look at some domains of cognition.

Direct Recall: Cognitive Training Concept #1: Here are some *direct recall* cognitive exercise examples to pair with focused movement:

- Recite the alphabet
- Recite the alphabet backwards (yes, we have people who do this perfectly)
- Name a country – have the client spell the country - then, spell it backwards
- Name a country and have the client name the capital of that country. Spell the capital and then spell it backwards
- Name their favorite movies. Have them name who starred in each movie
- Name favorite musicians or bands
- Name the USA presidents. Start with the current and name the predecessor of each as far back as they can
- Name vice presidents and do the same
- Do math equations
- Name every car make and model they have owned beginning with their present car and going back to their first car
- Name every country they have traveled to
- Name every major city they have traveled to
- Have them count forwards or backwards in increments (here are examples):
  - Count forwards incrementally (i.e., by 3's – 0, 3, 6, 9, 12, etc.)
  - Count backwards from 247 by 6's or 9's or any increment
  - While counting, change it up and cue the client to count backwards by 4's, 11's, 12's or any increment
  - Progress with more difficult counting, for example:

- Count backwards from 742 by 6's. Change it up at some point and count backwards by a different increment
- Change that up and have them count forward in various increments and then count backwards again
- Name body parts and spell each of them
- If they know anatomy, challenge them with anatomy questions
- Name and spell every kitchen appliance you can think of

Find out interests and hobbies and get creative with additional direct recall challenges. Here are examples of a few interests I have encountered:

- Cars
- Sports (teams, players, stats)
- Travel
- Cooking
- Photography
- Flowers
- Dogs
- Birds
- Music (musicians, songs, bands, etc.)
- Broadway shows
- Television shows
- Movies
- Astronomy
- Economics
- Art
- Gardening
- Hiking
- Reading

Spatial / Visuospatial Performance: Cognitive Training Concept #2

Remember, these can be done on their own, but visuospatial performance training will be more effective when paired with some type of focused movement.

"Take me from one place to another"

Example #1: Start at your current location. Have them imagine they are getting in their car and driving to their place of work, their home, their favorite restaurant, etc. Have them describe every part of the trip in the greatest detail possible:

- Street names
- Number of blocks or miles to the next turn
- Is there a stoplight or stop sign at each turn?
- Which direction will they go at each turn?
- What landmarks do they pass on the way?

Example #2: Obstacle course

Here is another exercise to train visuospatial and proprioceptive awareness.

- Set up an obstacle course
- Include objects to step *onto*
- Include objects to step *over* or to go *around*
    - i.e., cones and hurdles of various heights (perhaps 5-8 inches in height)
    - a wobble board
    - an airex pad
    - include some type of step-up platform or stairs
    - include a doorway
    - set up an agility ladder

Exercise #3: Hand-eye coordination

Adding a cognitive challenge during the games will stimulate the deeper brain:

- Play badminton
- Play basketball
- Play tennis
- Play volleyball
- Play ping pong (or table tennis)

Exercise #4: Virtual reality and augmented reality

If you have the tools available, try virtual reality or augmented reality gaming. Imaging shows that numerous areas of the brain light up and become active throughout the duration of the game. The more the brain lights up, the more likely new neural pathways are being created.

Decision Making / Reactive Training: Cognitive Training Concept #3:

In this concept of training, the primary goal involves speeding up reactive decision-making abilities. Here are a few examples:

- **Boxing**: using a heavy bag or with the coach wearing boxing mitts, the patient wearing boxing gloves, and the coach cueing each punch, try a few of the following reactive decision-making ideas:

  o When the coach cues "right" the client executes a punch using their right hand. When the coach cues "left" the client executes a punch using their left hand. If the coach is wearing mitts, establish a protocol for punching, for example: when the patient punches with their right hand, they are crossing over to hit the right mitt and vice versa for left side punches.

o Try putting colored tape or a colored sticker on the mitts. On my mitts, I have yellow tape on the left mitt and green tape on the right mitt. We now have the option of cueing the patient to hit *right, left, yellow, or green.*

o Progress this as follows: "everything the coach cues, the client does the opposite." For example, when the coach cues to hit *right*, the patient hits *left*. When the coach cues to hit *yellow*, the patient hits *green*, etc.

In each case, the client has to make the decision of which hand to punch with. Progressing to opposites creates a greater challenge as the client must *think, decide*, then *react* with the correct punch.

Try progressing this activity further. Here are some examples:

Enrich the proprioceptive environment by having the client stand on an airex pad, a wobble board, a Bosu *(bow sue)* ball, or some other somewhat unstable surface while boxing.

Add a cognitive challenge:

• with each punch, have the patient name a city they have traveled to
• have them tell you how to get from their current location to another location
• have them imagine they are going on vacation and ask them to name every item they would pack that begins with the letter "S" (i.e., sneakers, shoes, sweater, socks, etc.)

Agility dots: agility dots come in multiple colors, anywhere from 6-24 dots per package.

Set up a pathway of dots on the floor and try cueing your client in various ways, i.e.,

- Rotations: (Rotations are often a trigger for freezing of gait and increase fall risk. Rotation training is highly beneficial).

- With each step, have your client rotate to step on the next dot. They can take their time and do this at a comfortable pace
- Progress this by cueing each step, i.e.,
  o Right foot blue
  o Left foot red
  o Try cross over rotations. Have your patient cross the left leg in front of the right leg to rotate right and vice versa for the opposite direction, i.e.,
  o Cue *left foot blue*: the blue dot will be to the patients' right side. The left leg crosses in front of the right leg to step on the blue dot and vice versa for the other side

More examples can be found in part four and on the book support website.

Problem Solving: Cognitive Training Concept #4:

Parkour is a great way to fire up the brain and involves multiple cognitive training techniques that are implemented simultaneously, including spatial and decision making.

If you do not have access to a Parkour facility, try setting up an obstacle course.

When encountering an obstacle, the goal is to get to the other side. When the client (or traceur) reaches each obstacle, they will examine it *spatially* and then *decide* how to get to the other side (over it, under it, around it, or through it). Spatial and decision-making training are simultaneously activated, and the problem gets solved as they reach the other side of the obstacle. This makes for a great way to fire up the brain and create more new neural firing patterns.

DOMAINS OF MEMORY

We have recently expanded our programming to include additional domains of memory.

You'll find that certain domains of memory overlap with each other, as do certain domains of cognition and memory.

Working Memory

Let's look at two examples that can help to improve and expand working memory.

Example #1: Word List

Prior to beginning a focused movement, the coach will recite a list of words.

I would suggest starting with 4-6 words, i.e.,

- Boat
- Grapefruit
- Car
- Hammer
- Apple
- Chisel

Ask the client to recite the words back to you until they recite without errors.

Next, have the client begin some type of focused movement. During the movement, ask the client to recite the list of words.

Change cognitive focus and ask the client to perform another task during movement, i.e.,

- Name every kitchen appliance they can think of
- Name every body part they can think of
- Name their favorite movies

Return to the word list and ask the client to recite it again.

Add a second (interference) word list into the mix, i.e.,

- Highway
- Giraffe
- Pudding
- Hamster
- Canal
- Milk

Ask the client to repeat back to you. When they recite without errors, return to the first word list, and ask them to recite.

Later in the training session, return to the word lists and have the client recite again to the best of their ability, preferably during focused movement. It is always interesting to see what we remember later in the session.

This type of training should be individualized and appropriate for each client with respect to their working memory abilities.

Example #2: Logical Memory

We saw the Anna Thompson story in part two and here it is again. It is often used for logical memory testing. The story is presented orally. Patients are asked to freely recall the story immediately after it was read and again 25-35 minutes later. (Laura B. Zahodne, 2011)

Here is the Anna Thompson story. Read this to your patient:

"Anna Thompson of South Boston, employed as a cook in a school cafeteria, reported at the City Hall Station that she had been held up on State Street the night before and robbed of fifty-six dollars. She had four small children, the rent was due, and they had not eaten for two days. The police, touched by the woman's story, took up a collection for her." (Unknown, n.d.)

Now, have your patient recite the story back to you in as much detail as possible.

Next, read the story again and then have your patient begin some type of focused movement.

During focused movement, ask your patient to recite the story again in as much detail as possible. If they leave out details, that's fine, but don't help them.

The Anna Thompson story comes from a logical memory exam. This exam includes a specific set of tests given in a specific order with detailed instructions. A scoring system accompanies the exam. To access the entire exam and scoring system, visit the book support website.

Episodic memory

Episodic memory is a person's unique memory of a specific event, so it will be different from someone else's recollection of the same experience.

Forming an episodic memory involves several unique steps, each of which involves a separate system of the brain. The first step in the process is called encoding, a process that your brain goes through each time you form a new episodic memory. (Zimmermann, 2014)

Another step in the process of forming an episodic memory is called consolidation, which is basically baking the event into your long-term memory. This helps the memory become more strongly ingrained so that it is not lost if the brain suffers an impairment. Episodic memory can be affected by trauma, hydrocephalus, tumors, metabolic conditions such as Vitamin B1 deficiency, and neurological diseases such as Alzheimer's disease. (Zimmermann, 2014)

Some examples of episodic memory:

- Where you were and the people you were with when you found out about the 9/11 attacks

- Your most recent vacation

- The first time you flew in an airplane

- The details about how you learned of a relative's death

- Fearing water because you almost drowned as a child

- Your first day at college or a new job

- Attending a friend or relative's 50th anniversary party

- Your first time driving a car

Short-term memory

Short term memory involves recall of information for a relatively short time (such as a few seconds). But *short-term memory* is the primary bottleneck in human information processing. Only a few items—the usual estimate is seven, plus or minus two—can be held in mind at once, and the items are immediately subject to fading or being overwritten.

Examples include:

- Remembering a phone number just given to you

- Remembering a person(s) name(s) when you first meet them
- Remembering a list of words (such as the word list examples already given in this chapter).

Prospective memory

Prospective memory, which compiles one's intentions to act in a certain way in the future, has been described as "remembering to remember." The sorts of memories that fit into this category allow people to accomplish the tasks that they want to do or are supposed to do—but can't do immediately. (Staff, n.d.)Examples include:

- Remembering to take medications at night

- Buying a gift for a family member or friend's birthday

- Calling someone at a certain time

- Vote on Election Day

- Run specific errands

Explicit Memory

Explicit memory, also known as declarative memory, refers to memories involving personal experiences as well as factual information which we can consciously retrieve and intentionally articulate.

Recalling information from explicit memory involves some degree of conscious effort – information is consciously brought to mind and "declared."

For example, declarative knowledge involves "knowing that:"

- London is the capital of England
- Zebras are animals

- The date of your mom's birthday etc. (Perera, 2020)

Implicit Memory

Implicit memory, also known as unconscious memory or automatic memory, refers to perceptional and emotional unconscious memories which influence our behavior.

The impact which implicit memory has on our current behavior occurs without our conscious retrieval of memories. (Perera, 2020)

Hence, implicit memory enables our prior experiences to improve our performance of various tasks without our conscious and explicit awareness of such experiences.

The impact which implicit memory has on our current behavior occurs without our conscious retrieval of memories. (Perera, 2020)

Hence, implicit memory enables our prior experiences to improve our performance of various tasks without our conscious and explicit awareness of such experiences.

- **Procedural Learning**: Procedural memory is part of implicit memory that is responsible for knowing how to perform a of particular types of action, such as:
    - reading
    - typing
    - tying shoes
    - riding a bike

Procedural memories are automatically retrieved for the execution of procedures involved in both cognitive and motor skills. This enables task performance without the need for conscious control or attention. The association of procedural learning with muscle memory can make certain actions second nature (Bullemer, Nissen, & Willingham, 1989).

- **Priming**: Priming memory is a non-conscious form of human implicit memory concerned with perceptual identification of words and objects.

Priming can be associative, negative, positive, affective, conceptual, perceptual, repetitive, or semantic. The subtle effects which this complex psychological phenomenon encompasses can be employed to manipulate individual behavior. (Perera, 2020)

Priming memory can also be exercised as follows (using the first three "memory" words in the beginning of the chapter: cucumber, green, and pickle. If the patient doesn't remember the first word, "green" – perhaps give them a clue, such as:

- o What color is the grass?

Once they say GREEN, ask them to recall the next word (cucumber). Use a "priming" clue such as

- o It's a long and narrow green vegetable

Once they say "cucumber" – ask for the third word in the list. If they have difficulty with this, prime them with:

- o What can you make out of cucumbers?

They may say "salad." They're right but prime them further and give more clues until they give you the correct third word, "pickle."

Autobiographical memory

Autobiographical memory is arguably our most important type of memory. These are the memories of our lives. When you think about a memory, you are probably thinking of an autobiographical memory. This is long-term memory that pertains to the events that you yourself have witnessed. There are as many examples of autobiographical memory as there are events that can happen in one's life. (Harell, 2021)

Examples include:

- Your wedding
- The birth of a child
- Graduation day
- Receiving the award
- High school memories
- College memories
- Childhood memories

Flashbulb memory

A flashbulb memory is a highly vivid and detailed 'snapshot' of a moment in which a consequential, surprising, and emotionally arousing piece of news was learned. (Perera, Flashbulb Memory, 2021)

Examples include:

- Where were you on 9/11 when the planes hit the Twin Towers?
- Where were you when JFK was assassinated?
- Where were you when your favorite baseball team won the world series?

Semantic memory

Semantic memory is a category of long-term memory that involves the recollection of ideas, concepts and facts commonly regarded as general knowledge. Examples of semantic memory include factual information such as grammar and algebra. (Perera, Semantic Memory, 2020)

Examples of semantic memories include:

- Recalling that Albany of the capital of New York
- Recalling that July 4, 1776, is the date which the USA became independent
- Recalling the type of food people eat in Mexico
- Knowing that elephants and giraffes are both mammals (Perera, Semantic Memory, 2020).

A QUICK REVIEW BEFORE WE MOVE ON

Remember that it is our intention to improve movement, memory, cognition, and reaction time.

Combining one or more cognitive challenges during movement will help to improve movement and multitasking abilities.

Also remember the two-step process to maximize benefits to the brain:

- Hyper-focus
- Sleep

In the next chapter, you'll find a list of our favorite products along with descriptions and benefits of using each product.

Continue "stacking" with additional challenges

Combining exercises from the lists above allows for versatility and creativity in your programming, but let's take it a step or two further by adding more exercise modalities into the mix.

Hand-eye Coordination

Hand-eye coordination offers a multitude of training benefits and is a mainstay in our education and training sessions. A short list of exercises or games that we find beneficial include:

- Play catch with a ball (and try doing it while doing one of the movements listed in the beginning of this chapter)
- Play catch with a ball with letter and/or numbers on it (and try doing it while doing one of the movements listed in the beginning of this chapter)
- Play badminton
- Play basketball
- Play tennis
- Play volleyball
- Play ping pong (or table tennis)

These games and exercises offer numerous benefits to the *brain* and have the potential of helping to improve:

- Visuospatial awareness
- Reaction time
- Cardiovascular conditioning
- Dual-task and multi-tasking abilities
- Cognition

Infinity Walk

The Infinity Walk is an effective exercise to simultaneously activate the visual and vestibular systems and helps to increase activity between the right and left hemispheres of the brain.

Adding the addition of a cognitive exercise during the Infinity Walk will further increase brain activity.

We find this exercise helps to improve rotations (an action that often triggers freezing of gait and falls) and increases the automaticity of upper and lower body rotation/counter-rotation thus improving the body's overall coordination and endurance. (John C. Murray, n.d.)

Implementation:

- Place 2 small objects a few feet apart (6-8 feet apart)
- Beginning in the middle of the 2 objects, have your client begin walking around the objects in a "figure 8" pattern outside then inside the objects.
- Once your client feels comfortable with this movement, add educational visual materials i.e., picture cards, phonic cards, spelling words, sight words, math facts, etc. To do this, start the client in the center of the chairs with his/her back to the object of attention (flashcards, tv, etc.). As your client walks the pattern, he/she should never lose sight of the target.

Keeping sight of the target causes the head to turn (activating the vestibular system) and eyes to track (activating the visual system).

Chapter Summary

Moving and thinking at the same time is highly beneficial to improve multitasking abilities.

Adding additional challenges (stacking) such as hand-eye coordination or vestibular/visual activation will fire up more brain activity and further develop improved multitasking abilities.

Remember the most important steps to realize faster improvements:

- HYPERFOCUS during every exercise
- SLEEP (maximize your sleep potential with the steps outlined in chapter 5. SLEEP is where the brain solidifies the new neural firing pathways sparked during your exercises)
- Be mindful of safety
  - Challenge yourself, but don't kill yourself
  - Challenge yourself and push yourself beyond normal limits, but do it in the safest way possible to minimize fall risk

Chapter 9

Unique and Highly Effective Tools to Enhance Results

CLMBR

We like the CLMBR so much, we have three of them in our clinic! They are used more than any other pieces of equipment in our clinic, and for very good reasons.

The CLMBR offers a multitude of benefits for body and brain health. In fact, it is our experience that the CLMBR offers the *most* benefits for body and brain health.

The CLMBR offers a low impact, high performance, high intensity cardiovascular workout while also building strength in 86% of your muscles, including working skeletal muscle above the heart (a feature unique to climbing). Due to a higher VO2 max, the high output allows the body to continue burning fat and calories hours after the workout. (CLMBR, n.d.)

We know that an elevated heart rate causes the creation of neurochemicals in the brain, including BDNF (brain derived neurotrophic factor). This offers countless benefits to brain, including:

- Maintenance and integrity of the structure and health of brain cells

- The slowing or possible elimination of the death of dying brain cells

- Additional blood and oxygen to the brain

- Possible delay or elimination of brain related disease onset

The CLMBR movement emulates a vertical crawling pattern. This reciprocal arm-leg movement pattern causes the two hemispheres of the brain to communicate and work together more effectively.

In our experience, the CLMBR offers a one-of-a-kind, unique brain and body workout for that is unparalleled.

Learn more about CLMBR at: www.karlsterling.com

T2 Iso-Trainer

The T2 Iso-Trainer is changing the world of fitness by providing a single solution fitness tool that exceeds the capabilities of any other device on the planet. We especially love the isokinetic aspect of it.

As simple and compact as the device may appear, it is unmatched in its ability to not only replace single-function equipment like free weights, suspension trainers, resistance bands, and battle ropes, it exceeds their capabilities. (T2 Iso-Trainer, 2022)

Isokinetic exercise is defined as maximum effort under controlled speeds using accommodating variable resistance. This is a highly efficient and effective method for building strength!

Additionally, the contralateral action of the T2 Iso-Trainer causes the two hemispheres of the brain to work together in ways that cannot be realized using other strength training devices.

At the link provided below, you will see that during concentric movement, exercisers use the opposing limb to provide resistance.

This is the highest quality and most adaptable, versatile, portable, and affordable tool we have ever seen!

Learn more and order your T2 Iso-Trainer at:

www.karlsterling.com

Power Plate®

While there are a multitude of companies providing vibration products, I exclusively use Power Plate® products for any form of vibration therapy. They make a variety of vibration devices. and the quality of their products are unparalleled. See chapter 7 for details.

Learn more about PowerPlate at: www.karlsterling.com

BHOUT: The World's First Boxing Bag with a Brain

We know that boxing offers many benefits to the body and brain, including:

- Improved cardiovascular health

- Increased bone density through impact forces to the hands

- Hand-eye coordination (foot-eye coordination, too)

- Increased blood and oxygen to the brain

- Improved cognition, memory, and reaction time

Rather than using a standard boxing bag, we much prefer using the BHOUT boxing bag.

The BHOUT Bag is a boxing bag unlike all the others. Its multi-layered system guarantees the best impact feeling.

It is the world's first bag with a brain (i.e., a processor) that combines the impact information from the sensors on the body of the bag, with sensors in the docking station and the 3D computer vision from the camera, integrated by their Artificial Intelligence system. Altogether, it allows you to know what kind of strike you are delivering (punches, kicks, elbows, knees), how many times, where and how hard. Additionally, future software releases will allow for more data and information. (BHOUT, n.d.)

Every strike to the bag is tracked using the latest technology. You can personalize every training session and exercise in the manner that works best for you. Track your progress, earn badges, climb the ranks, and grow with BHOUT.

Exercise can feel like a constant battle of motivation and determination.

BHOUT has created an experience that helps you to get in the best shape of your life while learning a new skill. You will never want to miss a workout again.

Share your workouts with friends. Challenge and support each other. BHOUT offers the perfect combination of fitness, gaming, fun and connection. (BHOUT, n.d.)

Learn more about BHOUT at: www.karlsterling.com

BrainSpeed Ball

About the same size as a basketball (but much lighter), the BrainSpeed Ball is a staple of every session for all our clients.

It has the complete alphabet printed on it in addition to numbers 1 through 12.

Visit the book support website to see video demonstrations of the many cognitive exercises we do.

Learn more about the BrainSpeed Ball at:

www.karlsterling.com

Motion Guidance

This has quickly become another staple of our programming. This is a one-of-a-kind system offering countless benefits:

- Gain immediate visual feedback
- Improve posture
- Increase core strength
- Improve gait
- Activate visual and vestibular systems
- Joint rehabilitation

As of this writing, the Clinician Kit includes everything you need to set your clinic up with visual feedback, for any body part! The Clinic Kit comes with one green rechargeable laser (low level, 1mW power), 4 hygienic body straps (S,M,L,XL) which compliment any body part and easily clean between patients, and a variety of tracking mounts and targets. (Guidance, n.d.)

Here's a look at what you are getting:

- A Soft-Shell Case

- 1 Green Laser with Case and USB/Wall Charging Components

- 2 of Each Mounting Piece (Flat and Perpendicular)

- 1 Extra Large, 1 Large, 1 Medium, and 1 Small Hygienic Body Straps (Wipeable Material)

- 2 Suction Hooks and 4 Sticky Hooks

- A Double Sided Thick 3x5' Tracking Grid

- A Thin 4x4' "Maze and Clock" Hangable Grid

- 1 Colored Silicone Hangable "Circle Target" (Guidance, n.d.)

Learn more about Motion Guidance at: www.karlsterling.com

Alpha Champs Lateral Rebound Trainer

As a neuro rehabilitation specialist, I am always looking for the highest quality tools to help my patients with Parkinson's disease and other neurological disorders.

The AlphaChamp LRT is among the most innovative and effective tools to help our patients to reduce fall risk and improve balance, stability, agility, mobility, reflexes, reaction time, and quality of life.

The AlphaChamp LRT is a one-of-a-kind unique and versatile product that uses trampoline technology and provides options to do exercises that can't be done on a standard trampoline or any other surface.

Our patients LOVE the AlphaChamp LRT! They experience the unique benefits it offers and always look forward to using it.

Learn more about the AlphaChamp LRT at: www.karlsterling.com

BoBo

The BoBo balance board is another of our favorite tools. BoBo merges balance with gaming to provide a fun and challenging set of exercises for the body and brain.

With BoBo Health, common physical therapy exercises and tools turn into an interactive, gamified experience for improved patient engagement and increased rehabilitation rates. Easily measure progress and outcomes, track quality and quantity of movements and exercises, and personalize each and every program. (BoBo, n.d.)

Trainers and therapists: maintain a personal relationship with your patients while meeting rising demands for remote treatments and growing your patient base. Provide a seamless blend of in-person and remote treatment. (BoBo, n.d.)

Our patients and clients love that BoBo turns common rehabilitation training into motivating and challenging games that make exercising a fun and rewarding activity and therapy.

BoBo offers two versions of the board:

- BoBo PRO
- BoBo Wobbly (home use)

For details and to order your BoBo (and receive a 10% discount), visit:

www.karlsterling.com

Vitruvian

The Vitruvian Trainer+ is amazing! It's a real gym, generating resistance from **0-440lb (200kg)** of *digital weight.*

The Vitruvian Trainer+ uses artificial intelligence to adjust the weight to you in real time, giving you the optimal workout, always.

AI reads your motion 1000 times per second, loading the right weight for you in every moment. This literally puts the optimal resistance in your hands.

Whether you're feeling fired up or fatigued, the Trainer+ knows exactly when to increase or reduce the load (with every rep) to give you the best workout experience possible.

We love the machine for many reasons. It is smart, compact, highly versatile, and easily portable, which allows us to take it to house calls we do with many of our clients.

Learn more at: www.karlsterling.com

REAXING Products

REAXING Products are among our very favorite of all we use! As described on the REAXING website, REAXING is a philosophy of life and an innovative training methodology based on a patented technology. The innovation of this technology consists in delivering, during the motor gesture, sudden sensory impulses to force and/or encourage the user to react. From this technology was born a line of exclusive products with greater effectiveness than normal equipment and which thus allows to accelerate the training results. (REAXING, n.d.)

The REAXING methodology, also known as neuroreactive training, allows you to train the neuro motor response to the unpredictability, in an effective and diversified way, with the aim of increasing its speed and "dynamic competence." In synthesis, we could affirm that – as it was at the origins of the human movement – the brain supremacy has been re-established over muscles. (REAXING, n.d.)

In our clinic, we use the following REAXING products (with more products to come soon):

The REAX BOARD: The only board with the *Sudden Dynamic Impulses* technology. Each workout reaches the highest neuromuscular intensity level with endless training solutions. Standard exercises, performed under stable and predictable conditions, become unpredictable, effective, and much more intense: all the muscles involved during the exercise are activated and the focus must be kept high and steady. (REAXING, n.d.)

REAX LIGHTS PRO: A patented technology to improve motor skills, cognition, peripheral vision, and reactivity.

Reax Lights Pro is an integrated concept designed to develop interactive training programs, combinations of tasks and reflexes improvement.

The Reax Lights system is the only one that includes mobile satellites, walls and floors, as well as a complete range of accessories for an innovative cognitive training. (REAXING, n.d.)

FLUIBALL: FLUIBALL is the first medicine ball with a variable quantity of non-toxic colored fluid inside, turning any exercise into a truly high-intensive neuromuscular training. Its features make it suitable for sport, fitness, and rehab. It has a specific "warp and weft," which makes it nearly unbreakable, while keeping it soft and easy to handle. FLUIBALL is a resistant ball with a variable quantity of liquid inside. The weight varies according to the quantity of liquid, while the combination of air and fluid gives a kinetic effect to any movement, making it a one-of-a-kind product.

FLUIBALL is available in several weights and sizes. It goes from 500 grams to 12 kilos. Each weight is univocally identified by a specific color. (FLUIBALL, n.d.)

FLUIKETTLE: The Fluikettle is composed by a particular soft rubber that make it a unique piece of equipment: it can be shaken, grabbed, thrown, without any risks of damaging people or surfaces. Thanks to these features, it can be used in a club, in a studio or at home even with a nice and sophisticated floor. Unlike the traditional cast iron kettlebell, the Fluikettle contains a mixture of solid and fluid which turns every workout into a genuine neuromuscular training event which is much more effective. The special feeling and the soft rubber make every activity a pleasant and harmonic movement. Unlike the traditional cast iron product, the Fluikettle's special material guarantees comfort during the workout execution because it is soft on the person.

Learn more about these and other REAXING products at: www.karlsterling.com

The Breath Belt

This is another game changing product. The Breath Belt is a one-of-a-kind diaphragmatic breath training tool that activates the gluteal muscles. The non-stop, tactile diaphragmatic breath cues alleviate muscles and fascial restriction of the abdominal muscles, allows the Psoas and Quadratus Lumborum Muscles to function with less restriction. (Belt, n.d.)

Learn more about The Breath Belt at: www.karlsterling.com

HandEyeBody

The HandEyeBody Coordination Charts are a staple of our training sessions with every patient in every session.

Empower people of all abilities to move with a level of confidence they've never known before.

HandEyeBody Coordination Charts are fun and functional tools that you can print & implement immediately to help your students, clients, and athletes unlock physical and mental abilities they never knew they had. And you'll have a lot of fun too!

The HandEyeBody Coordination Power Pack & Exercise Library will transform how you teach essential functional skills, including hand-eye coordination, multi-tasking, visual tracking, fine motor control, reaction speed, memory and concentration, sensory processing, and more! (HandEyeBody, n.d.)

Learn more at: www.karlsterling.com

Step and Connect / Balance Matters®

Balance Matters® is an evaluation and treatment system that includes a measuring tool on the mats used for the assessment of specific gait parameters, namely step length and step width. Evaluation findings can be directly transferred to treatment and be used to establish objective monitoring of progress. Multisensory feedback tests and challenges the sensory systems for balance is provided through varied textured footprints, auditory feedback, and varied foam densities. Qualified healthcare professionals assess an individual's balance and gait to determine if the area(s) of deficits are in anticipatory postural adjustments, dynamic gait, sensory orientation, equilibrium strategies, or a combination of the above. Once the area(s) of balance dysfunction are identified, a customized objective program is created to improve balance and gait. (Connect, n.d.)

This is another of our very favorite products we use with every patient in every session.

Core-Tex Sit

Core-Tex Sit saves your lower back by creating a variable sitting environment.

The patented motion allows for a controlled, dynamic sitting experience that benefits your lower back, hips, core, and pelvic floor. Much more than just "anti-slouching" or core work, Core-Tex Sit dissipates stress on muscles and joints with subtle changes in position.

- Provides relief and prevents stress from accumulating on the lower back.
- Strengthens abdominal muscles and lower back while sitting.
- Great for posture and improved focus while working.
- Easy to use: Simply place Core-Tex Sit on your favorite firm chair and sit on it. No assembly or maintenance required. (Sit, n.d.)

Learn more at: www.karlsterling.com

Vision Sticks

The Vision Sticks are a great system to raise the potential of your sensory neurons and activate your brain in just 5 minutes of training. (Lococo, n.d.)

One of the most important parts of the body is the Visual System. It is a primary way to receive external information trigging millions of neuronal cells and activating all of your brain.

Learn more about Vision Sticks at: www.karlsterling.com

AIR RELAX

Many of the tools we use, including the AIR RELAX BOOTS, were originally intended for use by athletes. If you think about it, we are ALL athletes to some degree. Hence, we find the AIR RELAX BOOTS to be highly effective for all of our patients.

Athletic recovery is as important as training and nutrition.

Exercise is stress and, while it does provide lasting physical and psychological benefits, it also creates traumas or microtears in your soft tissue, specifically your muscles. This can lead to soreness and pain. An imbalance caused by overly intensive training and inadequate recovery will not only lead to injury but also to less effective training sessions.

There are many recovery methods available to athletes nowadays. The ones available to anyone are sleep and rest days. Yet many athletes like to take a more active approach to their recovery.

AIR RELAX RECOVERY BOOTS AND RECOVERY

Compression devices were once only for the exclusive use of patients with serious muscular and circulatory disorders such as lymphedema, venous insufficiency and P.A.D. Today, Recovery systems are used by sports teams, universities, physical therapists, and professional athletes to improve recovery time and enhance their training.

"Compression garments add external pressure. Blood can easily pool in the extremities, especially in the lower limbs due to gravity," writes exercise physiologist Ross Hamilton in his guide for recovery.

"The extra compression helps squeeze the blood out of the muscles and back to the lungs and heart. This allows fresh oxygenated blood to replace it."

Its benefits are said to include:

- Improved blood circulation
- Boost lymphatic fluid movement (reduce potential swollen legs/feet)
- Removal of lactic acid (reduce muscle fatigue)
- Improved flexibility
- Recovery stimulation
- Boost oxygen distribution

This is backed by research: a 2017 study found that external pneumatic compression mitigated a reduction in flexibility and pressure-to-pain threshold (the minimum force applied which induces pain), as well as reduced select skeletal muscle oxidative stress and proteolysis markers during recovery from heavy resistance exercise.

Another study concluded that peristaltic pulse dynamic compression is a promising means of accelerating and enhancing recovery after the normal aggressive training that occurs in Olympic and aspiring Olympic athletes. (RELAX, n.d.)

Additionally, we find the boots to be effective in temporarily reducing rigidity cause by Parkinson's.

Learn more at: www.karlsterling.com

RockTape

Kinesiology tape is powerful sensory input tool we find to be very effective. It is a favorite among live workshop attendees and with our clients, as well. As we know, people with PD tend to have a forward posture which leads to less-than-optimal movement and an increased risk of falling. RockTape is my personal favorite brand of kinesiology tape. It sticks well and is the most durable tape I have used.

Visit their website at: www.karlsterling.com

Stick Mobility

We use the Stick Mobility training system to improve flexibility, strength, and coordination.

The system combines joint mobilization, strength training, and active stretching to increase performance, reduce risk of injury, and accelerate recovery.

The exercises implement custom-designed Training Sticks as tools to improve range of motion, muscle activation, coordination, and body awareness to build a strong foundation for better movement.

The Stick Mobility system is based on the scientific principles of leverage, stability, feedback, irradiation, isometrics, and coordination.

Learn more at: www.karlsterling.com

HidrateSpark

I was introduced to HidrateSpark products at the 2022 Miami Beach IHRSA conference. Let me just say – they make super high-quality bottles that help to track hydration!

The average age of our patient population at my clinic is 81 years old. In general, and for a number of reasons, we find that this population has difficulty staying hydrated. The HidrateSpark is a great system to help keep you adequately hydrated!

HidrateSpark PRO is our bottle of choice. It is the world's smartest water bottle ever created. Available in stainless steel vacuum insulated material, it keeps drinks cold up to 24 hours in a lightweight, shatter and odor resistant Tritan ™ plastic. The LED smart sensor "puck" glows to remind you when it's time to drink and tracks your water intake by syncing via Bluetooth to the HidrateSpark App. Choose from 3 sizes and 2 lid options and make it your own with custom glow colors in the app. (HidrateSpark, n.d.)

Learn more at: www.karlsterling.com

ElectroSkip

ElectroSkip™ is an amazing tool we use to help improve gait. It works like this: sensors are placed under toes and heels. Wireless transmitters attach to the top of each foot. Your steps send a signal to a USB receiver that is converted into MIDI musical notes and beats by the computer. ElectroSkip™ kernel software allows you to remotely adjust the pressure sensitivity of the sensors.

ElectroSkip™ is one-of-a-kind and truly a new platform. Use it sitting, standing, skipping, and running. Generate your own beats from your sneaks! Whether you're a Tapper or Rapper, ElectroSkip™ gives you digital tap-dancing shoes, a MIDI compatible link to the world of electronic music, and a totally fluid way of generating loop-based music or adding a dynamic track over preexisting songs.

Learn more at: www.karlsterling.com

Urban Poling

Walking sticks/poles have been around for a long time. We exclusively use and recommend Urban poling product.

Urban poling (also known as Nordic walking)—think cross-country skiing without the skis—has toning, calorie-burning and posture benefits that have made it popular in Europe for decades and a new workout favorite in Canada. Just grab your poles and go—no need for a pricey spandex outfit or a fancy gym membership!

Urban poling offers many benefits including:

- Increased stability and mobility
- Core strengthening
- Improved posture

- Improved walking velocity

Learn more at: www.karlsterling.com

Vivo Barefoot

I am very particular about what I wear on my feet, and I wear barefoot shoes all the time.

I have tried every brand of barefoot shoe on the market (that I know of), and I exclusively wear only ONE brand: Vivobarefoot Shoes.

They are the most comfortable and durable I have ever owned. I have been wearing the same pair for 18 months and they are nowhere near worn out. I am very active, and I move a LOT every day. All other brands of barefoot shoes I tried have been completely worn out in 3-4 months. Vivobarefoot is the only brand I will wear.

The human foot is a biomechanical masterpiece; when left to its own devices it can thrive doing everything from walking and running to jumping and dancing, but by cramming it in a modern shoe - cushioned, narrow, and rigid - negates its natural strength and function. Our feet are our foundation connecting us to the earth, they should not be compromised.

All Vivobarefoot footwear is designed to be Wide, Thin and Flexible: as close to barefoot as possible. They promote your foot's natural strength and movement, allowing you to feel the ground beneath your feet.

There is a powerful sensory connection between the feet and the brain and thus, our movement and place in the world. A Vivobarefoot shoe reconnects you to the world around you, literally bringing you closer to nature.

Learn more at: www.karlsterling.com

StrongBoard Balance

StrongBoard Balance is unlike any other balance board in the industry, and it is the balance board of our choice in our clinic.

MULTI SPRING TECHNOLOGY™ works with your body to deliver the perfect amount of stimulation to keep your core musculature and stabilizing muscles engaged and contracted, while training your central nervous system, improving posture, proprioception, and reaction time.

Learn more at: www.karlsterling.com

OUR FAVORITE APPS:

Clock Yourself

Clock Yourself is a brain game that moves you. It combines cognitive and physical challenges into a brain game that makes you think on your feet.

The Clock Yourself concept originated in neurological rehabilitation. Now, anyone can use it to harness their neuroplasticity.

Clock Yourself in unapologetically low-tech and versatile in design, which is why it is popular with elite athletes, stroke survivors, and everyone in-between. (Yourself, n.d.)

Learn more at: www.karlsterling.com

Quizlet

Quizlet is a study set creation tool for students and teachers that gives lots of freedom to create. Quizlet is a fantastic tool for teachers to create quizzes for in-person and remote learning that makes building and assessing quick and easy.

It is versatile enough to offer adaptive, customized cognitive and memory training for each of our patients.

Learn more at: www.karlsterling.com

BrainHQ

BrainHQ is your online headquarters for working out your brain. Think of it as a personal gym, where you exercise your memory, attention, brain speed, people skills, intelligence, and navigation instead of your abs, delts, and quads. Just as our bodies require care and exercise over the course of life, so do our brains.

This is among our very favorite apps for training the brain!

Learn more at: www.karlsterling.com

Part Two

Inspiring Stories

Words from director of Parkinson's Si buko Uganda, Kabugo Hannington

My name is Kabugo Hannington. I am a food scientist with a bachelor's degree in food processing technology. I work with the Capital city authority of Uganda (KAMPALA CAPITAL CITY AUTHORITY) as a food and beverage supervisor, and I am the country director of Parkinson's Si buko Uganda (Parkinson's is not witchcraft).

My mom died many years ago because she had Parkinson's. My dad took us with him away from our mom and started renting a one-bedroom house because he never wanted us to get Parkinson's. He thought PD was contagious. He thought that if we stayed too close to his wife we too could get the disease. My mom suffered but she too welcomed the idea of leaving her alone because she wanted to save us from contracting Parkinson's.

It was a very sad moment of our lives leaving our dear mom in the house alone with all the PD stigmatisms. I thought "who's going to be helping her?" She never had any PD knowledge or medications. People who could give her food and water would just push her a plate with a stick because they would fear direct contact with her.

The time came when I couldn't hold my sadness and sorrow anymore because I always thought of my mom and how she was coping with the hardest situation of her life. I sneaked out of our rented apartment whenever my dad would go to work, and I would go to see my mom. The first day seeing her I couldn't believe the suffering she was going through. I just ran to her, hugged her, and told her, "Mom I love you and all will be all right now that I'm here." She cried and told me not to ever contact her because I will get the disease (PD). I boldly told her, "Mom, getting your disease through hugging - I'll be so

happy to have it for the rest of my life." As long as it's your disease, trust me, you can't send me away." I would insist to hug her always.

Seeing my mom suffer to death with no one close to her was so painful. She had no one; not her husband, not my sisters, none of her family members, and community all running away from her and calling her a witch while laughing at her because she's cursed. They believed that's why she has PD. Yet, to date after hugging my mom I have never gotten PD. That brought up something in my mind to let no one suffer my mom's way and it's the reason I started Parkinson's Si buko Uganda to let everyone know that PD isn't witchcraft or a curse. It's a science and it is a disease that one can live with.

Why would one suffer? Why wouldn't one know the truth about PD and why wouldn't one have access to medications? That's my goal and it's the reason we have this organization.

I thank Karl Sterling who laid a great foundation on this organization and giving me this opportunity to share my story to the world and changing people's lives every day. I thank Sherryl Klingelhofer my director, Omotola Thomas, Gavin Mogan, Russ Parker, and everyone who has been helping us to let everyone know about Parkinson's and to dispel that myth that PD is not witchcraft.

May God bless you all.

In my last visit to my Neurologist, I asked him how my PD has progressed in this last 7 years that I have been his patient. He told me progression is minimum. He thinks that I have a good and optimistic attitude and exercise has been what has helped me. I feel excellent! I have a normal and active life. I exercise and have a lot of energy. I just did what we all should do: exercise, have balanced and healthy diet, get adequate rest, smile, and do things that make you happy.

Please don't wait to get sick or until you are in a difficult situation in life.

Although it's not always been like this, at first, I felt sad because in his examinations I noticed all the movements and easy tasks I was unable to do and just didn't understand why.

He asked me about my family health background, so I asked my parents and other family members, and there was no one else with PD. It took me time to understand. I was slow in all my movements, had problems with stability and coordination, and people couldn't read my writing. I just cried and said, "when did this happen?"

I decided to leave my job because I didn't want additional stress in my life. I just wanted to try to do something about my PD. I had no information, no therapy, there was nothing for me.

My family always supported me 100% and more, but just didn't know how to help.

I did research and went to a public rehab center. I am pleased to tell you that exercise changed my life. I learned that I could do something about it. I attended the rehab center for several years. It was not easy, but I never stopped trying. I received excellent treatment there. We worked on physical and occupational therapies.

I have worked really hard on physical rehabilitation in public and private institutions here where I live, in Nuevo Laredo, Mexico. We are on the border with Laredo, Texas.

Both public and private rehab institutions signed me out. I really felt good and safe with them. They told me I was ready and able to enroll in a normal class and they recommended walking, swimming, yoga, bike riding, and everything that has to do with movement.

Now my doctor always asks me, how are you doing? How has Parkinson changed your life? And I tell him I am happier now! Of course, I don't like Parkinson's in my life, but I just learned to change my perception and enjoy everything it offers.

In one of my visits to the doctor, I asked him, is there something more I can do, more therapies, more information? He said look up and contact Karl Sterling, and so I did. I attended a workshop in Austin, Texas and since then I just keep on learning about what PD is and what can I do to be better.

I am 47 years old now and I've learned that not everything is Parkinson's. I do my best to try do understand what I feel. I've learned to observe and know my body and it has helped me to keep on moving!

I have lots of energy and Parkinson's symptoms have reduced significantly with exercise, yoga, meditation, and following my doctor's treatment and recommendations,

Parkinson doesn't define who we are, always remember that!

SMILE AND KEEP ON MOVING!

Besides doing home chores, I practice yoga and meditation on a daily basis. I also enjoy walking, running a bit, swimming, bicycling outdoors, and traveling (my very favorite). Recently I am doing acrylic painting in canvas. It helps my mind to be free. I just focus on my painting, and I love to dance and sing, too. I am also a community volunteer for cancer fundraising and other social causes. I feel I have a lot to offer as a person and an active community member. I have my own boutique (girls and ladies' clothes and accessories). I help my parents with lots of love and patience, and best of all, I enjoy my favorite roles in life: being a mom and wife. I am so happy and feel so blessed.

All of these activities make me feel that life is beautiful and even with Parkinson's, I want to enjoy every single moment with the ones I love, my family and friends.

PARKINSON'S AND COVID19

When all of this started, I said to myself, I have worked really hard retraining my body, I am currently working on retraining my mind, I thought that by following safety regulations I would be ok. And I was, for the first three months. I practiced meditation and yoga in my house, adapting a nice environment for it. After the third month I felt like an earthquake, or a tsunami was contained inside my body. What is happening? I had dedicated time observing myself. I thought I knew where I was standing, and all of these new emotions, because of social distance and restrictions, did not help me at all. I started doing more exercise, painting on canvas, and learned to use a sewing machine to make face coverings and donated them to private and public hospitals. I needed to somehow help from home, and so we did.

I helped my community, and I kept my mind busy for a while. Our brain is very powerful and in my case and because of less dopamine production, it affects my movement. So, all of this activity of creating and working with my hands really helped. I noticed that if I felt happy, my PD symptoms would be much less.

I feel happy and blessed because I am able to move, speak and do everything on my own. I thank God for all of these blessings.

I have been recently invited to participate in a private group in Facebook "Empowering persons with Parkinson's," there we share and learn together:

- Education in Parkinson's
- Respiration
- Movement
- Benefits of music and rhythms, among many others.

It's free, and for all patients and caregivers in Mexico. I serve as moderator, translator, and sharing my testimony always giving the best of me, it makes me feel empowered.

I never imagined that in the middle of a Pandemic and with my own issues, I was going to be able to serve others by listening to them, by sharing, by learning, dancing, enjoying together, all of this online with the zoom app.

Life is short, and we should value that and be always grateful.

Smile more, enjoy life!

HOW HAS MY PARKINSON'S AFFECTED MY FAMILY?

The word PARKINSON'S really caused on impact on me. When I told my husband, parents, and sisters, they were worried and didn't know how to help. I waited some years to tell my kids when they could understand better.

A few days ago, at home, I asked them, can you all share with me how has my PD affected you, if it has?

My daughter and son, 20 and 17 years old, told me that at first, they worried, but they have seen all my efforts and work I've done to be better. They have learned to be patient and understanding with me and with other people in a difficult situation, not only PD fighters.

And to my husband, who is the person that has lived along with me and my PD, I really appreciate all your support, your love, and your patience. I appreciate you believing in me when I told you, "I have decided to do something about this, I'll fight back against PD." And so, we did.

Thank you, Karl, for inviting me to collaborate in your book. I am honored that you considered me. I hope it helps other people with PD or another situation they are going through.

I would like to express my gratitude to my LIFE TEAM:

- MY FAMILY: for your love and support, you are my strength and happiness and the reason to keep on moving!
- MY NEUROLOGIST AND DEAR FRIEND: I have no words to express my appreciation for all your attentions to my person. Not only are you my doctor, you are my friend. Thank you!
- MY THERAPISTS: who have been with me since day one in rehab. Thank you for your patience and friendship.
- MY LOTS OF FRIENDS: for always having the perfect words to make me feel better and for seeing me for who I really am. I love each and every one of you.

Most of all, I want to thank God for giving me the strength and for surrounding me with all of these great people I mentioned. Thank you Lord for the many and wonderful blessings I receive form you.

And I just want to add, SMILE MORE, LAUGH, LOVE, ENJOY LIFE!

Thanks again Karl for letting me share my PD testimony!

See you in the next workshop!

LAURA OLMOS, June 28, 2020

Words from PD fighter, Russ Parker

Caring and Sharing

It is mid-2014 and I am all settled in as a personal trainer at the local YMCA. I was happy with my client load and was lucky, too that all my clients were a pleasure to work with. Most of my clients were middle aged, looking to stay fit, lose some weight and avoid/relieve aches and pains.

My client Joel was the first client I ever worked with that had more than just some aches and pains. Joel has Multiple Sclerosis. I knew a little about MS from research I had done and from information I received as part of an MS fundraising race that I competed in. Joel's MS symptoms were fortunately not severely debilitating, but MS is no picnic and symptom flare-ups could arise at any time. Joel had a positive, "can do" attitude about his condition, which I admired. There were a few issues he wanted to address, and he also wanted help with his strength training routine.

His first training session with me turned out to be a very rewarding day for both of us. After assessing his condition, I learned that one issue he had was he could barely lift his left leg off the ground, while his right leg was totally fine. I had a couple of ideas in my head to try and get that left leg working better. The first idea did not work. Then I had him perform an exercise that forced his hip into flexion with very gentle assistance using the platform of the assisted pull-up machine to provide. While the assistance help put his leg through the full range of motion, some effort was still needed on his part. The combination was just the right mix, which stimulated neuromuscular activation through the full range of motion. After completing the exercise, Joel could now raise his left foot off the ground and flex his hip into a normal range of motion.

During the rest of the session, he was periodically lifting his foot off the ground, looking amazed at his newfound range of motion. I reflected on it later that day and it brought tears of joy to my eyes being happy for Joel and grateful for the opportunity to make a difference in someone's life. It also reinforced my belief that the human body is more resilient than people give it credit for and that thinking outside the box can open the door to bringing about change that exceeds the expectation of the mainstream. I also realized how fortunate I was. For people with MS, some days just getting out of bed is a struggle and I was lucky to be living an active life without such severe struggles. These thoughts and emotions that I experienced that day, foretold how within the next couple of years I indeed would become all too familiar with struggles from having a debilitating movement disorder and how that also developed into an opportunity to help others.

Fast forward a little more than one year later to August 2015, I had been enjoying my first few years in my new favorite sport of running. I had to shut down my running though because I was having recurring pain problems in my right hip, lower back and feeling very stiff in general. I didn't want to injure myself, so I worked on healing. After getting only some relief from various treatments and exercise, I finally saw a neurologist and was diagnosed with Parkinson's Disease, in April 2016.

From my symptoms and research, I knew for several months that PD diagnosis was a possibility. Being a positive person, I was prepared to accept a PD diagnosis and move forward. I saw this as a challenge and an opportunity. I pledged to friends and family that I would

136

fight this disease with every ounce of my being. I was determined to learn as much as I could about fighting this disease not just to help myself, but to help others. I knew how important exercise was in helping to fight PD. I planned on leveraging my experience as a trainer, my positive attitude and determination to leave no stone unturned to help and inspire others. My past experiences helping clients move better and now this PD diagnosis convinced me that my calling was to specialize in exclusively training people with Parkinson's Disease and other movement disorders.

My goal was to not only train people with Parkinson's, but to help educate others on the importance of exercise and help empower people with PD with knowledge to help themselves beyond just medication. Ramping up my knowledge on human movement, movement disorders and neuro-rehabilitation techniques would help me and others slow progression of symptoms and possibly slow disease progression. To give myself as much opportunity as possible to learn, I aggressively pursued education through classes, workshops, conferences etc. I also ramped up my networking efforts interacting online and in person with people in the PD community and with other professionals. Also, my own experiences with PD and observing my clients with PD served as another educational experience. As a person with PD, I have become a walking test lab for getting real time feedback on the effectiveness of various approaches to fighting symptoms and disease progression. While everyone has their variation of the disease and how it impacts them, my situation provides me with a high level of understanding of what my PD clients are going through.

Despite the frustrations that come with being a person with Parkinson's, the experiences I have had, what I have learned, and friends I have made has enriched my life beyond my wildest imagination. Inspiration, passion, sharing, and mutual support permeates the amazing group of people that is the Parkinson's community. I owe a debt of gratitude to my fellow PD fighters and all the professionals and caregivers.

I have been training, coaching, and educating people with PD for almost three years now. One of the things that all my clients have in common that impresses me is that they chose a path to commit to doing more than address the symptoms and progression of Parkinson's disease than just take medication. They have learned that exercise is beneficial in helping improve quality of life in addition to what medications do and were willing to take on exercise as a treatment. Even though none of them are particularly exercise enthusiasts and often suffered from lack of energy, they are willing to put their faith in me and give it their best shot. I commend them for that. It has been a challenge, but I feel I have had a positive impact on my client's quality of life, especially considering the limited amount of time I spend with them. This disease manifests itself in many ways not just from person to person but varies from day to day. I have grown as a trainer and a person in the last few years in ways that may not have happened if I didn't have PD. I learned the importance of knowing the intricacies of human movement, how the brain, nervous systems and many other systems in the human body affect each other. This better enabled me to know how to adapt, so that positive changes resulting in better movement could occur. I also have learned to have a higher appreciation of the importance of play and fun in our life.

Purposeful movement is important, but I learned that adding a dose of fun can be like a turbo boost to the brain that helps one's movement shift to a higher gear - like the time that my client Bob was struggling to walk, and I decided to throw some music into the mix. Bob is in his 80's so I figured he'd appreciate some Frank Sinatra. As the song "You Make Me Feel So Young" was playing, his posture and gait immediately improved, and he was walking with confidence (and singing along, too). As I was walking with him, I sang along too and was wishing I had a video of that feelgood moment. With my client Rocco, I found out he enjoyed competing in different sports, so I make sure I periodically add in sports movements like throwing, catching, boxing, golfing etc. These are a couple of examples of the joy and satisfaction that I experience from working with people with PD. I also feel a special bond with them, having PD myself. They appreciate the fact that I treat them not like people who are disabled or old, but an empowered partner in a relationship with me. Their trust in me and their kindness towards me makes me feel good about myself and what I am doing. I believe in the goodness of people and welcome every opportunity to establish caring and sharing relationships.

One of my most challenging and most inspirational clients is Gary. He is truly amazing! Gary has Progressive Supranuclear Palsy (PSP) which is classified as a Parkinson's Plus disease. It progresses much faster than PD, symptoms are more intense and harder to control and along with that, fall risk is increased. Gary needs to use a walker when moving about the house. But when he works with me, we work on walking, handling freezing and festination in his walking gait, all without a walker.

Gary will go to whatever lengths it takes to fight PSP and slow symptom progression. The disease progresses very quickly and when using exercise as a treatment, if you don't take the use it or lose it approach from the start, symptom progression can accelerate, and the person becomes severely disabled only a few years after diagnosis. Motor symptoms like severe instability, festination of gait (rapid uncontrollable small steps) and freezing of gait can get worse very rapidly without intervention along with other non-motor symptoms like swallowing and vision problems. Medications have minimal effect. Gary was initially diagnosed with Parkinson's Disease and started right away with exercise joining a Rock Steady Boxing class, walking every day on the treadmill, and strength training. Even with all that, PSP was still impacting his movement and he was already a big fall risk and I'm sorry to say, he has fallen many times. I spot him very closely, but he fell a few times with me. Nothing too bad, but I still of course feel bad about it. The thing is, many other people in the same position as him would not be a fall risk at this point. But that is because they would have already deteriorated to the point of being wheelchair bound. Gary amazingly has avoided that fate. His bravery and relentless attitude to never give up is bringing tears to my eyes as I write this. This has been a tough fight and one day the progressive nature of PSP will perhaps be too much for him, but not today. I am glad that I have been able to help this amazing man carry on to this point.

This is where my pursuit of education came in handy. I needed every trick in the book to help Gary with his gait and instability problems. I learned a lot of cool stuff from human movement experts over the last few years. The foundation of my approach is influenced the most by everything I learned from my dear friend Karl Sterling and his Parkinson's Regeneration Training workshops, his book, and online resources. I am now part of Karl's presentation team that also includes my friends Alison Klaum and Ruben Artavia who am also grateful to know.

I worked with Gary a lot on fall prevention, nervous system activation, multitasking and cognitive training techniques that I had learned. Through specific targeted training and some trial and error I was able to help him with his gait and balance problems and was also able to restore his ability to walk on the treadmill which he lost for a brief period. The amazing thing is how Gary pushes himself competitively through a training session. I can't begin to describe how difficult this must be with all the symptoms he has. Imagine someone constantly bumping you while you are trying to walk, ball bearings randomly imbedded in the soles of your shoes, so you are slipping and sliding out of control, wearing glasses that distort your vision, the floor occasionally moving like a merry-go-round, being zapped with a taser, and wearing clothes two sizes too small that constrict your movement. O.K., this description may sound a bit dramatic, but it is meant to emphasize the amazing resilience of Gary as much as it is a description of awful symptoms. He is my hero. I know Gary will never quit and he inspires me to continue relentlessly in my own fight against Parkinson's Disease, to help my fellow PD fighters and be inspired by many others as well.

My life has changed a lot since being diagnosed with Parkinson's Disease. Some of those changes are not pleasant, but I choose to focus on the positive. Going into this fight as a positive person, I felt I had what it takes to meet this challenge. That positive attitude has certainly helped, but I totally underestimated the powerful, inspirational impact that so many people would have on me. I am a better person because of the influence of many wonderful people from the new people I have met to my family and friends. I will do my best to rise up against adversity and take as many as I can along for the ride.

Words from caregiver, Donna Parker

A Caregiver's Tale of Two Parkinson's Journeys

When my husband, Russ, was first diagnosed with Parkinson's Disease, I won't say I didn't face it with some degree of trepidation and fear. It had crossed my mind that the symptoms he had been experiencing were due to Parkinson's, but I put it out of my mind hoping they were due injuries brought on by his active lifestyle.

I had been here before. I had already seen up close how Parkinson's Disease could disrupt one's life. My mother had been diagnosed with Parkinson's some 20 years earlier and we had watched her decline over a 10-year period to the point where she was bedridden and spending her days watching TV and sleeping. Her short-term memory was impaired, and she had broken both hips mostly because she didn't remember not to get up and walk without assistance. In addition, due to her memory issues, rehab was difficult. It was hard for her to remember from one day to the next what the physical therapists had done with her the day before and how to safely stand and walk using her walker.

My dad was her primary caregiver for years. As is often the case, he sacrificed his own health to lovingly care for her. My sister and I tried to assist as much as possible and he finally agreed to get some outside help. But as often happens, PD had taken its toll on him, and he died a few years later.

At this point, my sister and I became mom's primary caregivers continuing to care for my mom with the same deep love and maintaining the same course of action that the doctors had previously prescribed. We followed the doctors' orders but never really questioned their recommended treatment, researched the disease, or investigated therapies that might potentially be helpful or bring some relief.

I never really remember mom being "on" after taking her meds. I think now that maybe the dosage wasn't quite right or perhaps, she was eating too close to each dose and her meals were interfering with the effect of the meds but none of these things occurred to me at the time. I didn't know how much better she should feel after taking her meds – these were only things I learned after Russ was diagnosed. We knew that exercise helped her, but she was difficult to motivate. We didn't press the issue.

We wanted to keep mom in her home. We knew she wouldn't do well in a nursing home after seeing how she dealt with her time in rehab, so our main concern became finding responsible and compassionate caregivers to look after her. This became a source of stress especially since we couldn't be there all the time to monitor her care. We were finally able to find a caregiver who mom seemed comfortable and happy with. She did her best to feed mom healthy meals and keep her engaged and moving as much as possible.

But, in the end, it seemed mom had given up hope. The person who had cared for so many sick relatives and friends all her life was now in need of that same loving care, and she was not ready to fight the disease that had overcome her.

So, when Russ was diagnosed with the same disease, I wondered what life ahead would hold. I knew our children and I would be there for him no matter what, but we all wanted so much more for him. He was diagnosed at a much younger age than my mom and he always brought so much fun and laughter into our lives. He had retired from a long career in Information Technology just a few years prior and had started a second career as a Personal Trainer hoping to help others maintain the same healthy lifestyle he had practiced for so many years. We looked forward to spending many happy years together traveling and dancing (one of our favorite pastimes). Our children, Carrie, and Chris didn't really remember much about my mom and her feisty personality before Parkinson's (she had become very quiet and docile) so they were also worried about their dad's future. I felt it was up to me to keep the family optimistic about his future, so I tried to remain positive and keep things light.

But Russ had a very different approach than my mom in dealing with his diagnosis. He wasn't going to let it get the better of him. He dove into researching the disease and what could be done to delay its progression. He sought out experts who had done detailed studies and, in addition to the standard meds, recommended dietary changes, exercise for both mind and body and a variety of supplements that had been proven to help with symptoms and even slow the progression of the disease. He networked and joined support groups to gather as much information as he could. Russ took complete control of his treatment always questioning and never taking anything at face value.

From the beginning, I saw my primary role as a caregiver as being a supportive partner providing help and encouragement in any way possible. I told him early on to concentrate on the fight he had ahead of him and not to worry about anything else. For now, that has meant taking on many of the household responsibilities that were previously his. It can be overwhelming at times but it's well worth it if it helps him to maintain the daily routine that keeps his symptoms under control. I've even found some of the tasks like gardening help me to focus and relax. During the early years in our home, Russ had planted a beautiful garden in our yard. With his father's advice and an inherited green thumb, he worked hard to make our yard a peaceful haven. Then he seemed to lose interest and things started to become overgrown. As I look back, this may have been brought on by the onset of his Parkinson's Disease. With his help, I'm trying to regain control of the garden, eliminating the weeds and vines that have taken over, learning to prune and shape the many bushes he planted, and planting new flowers where the ones he had planted have long since disappeared. I often ask his advice about what should go where (does a particular plant or bush need sun or shade, dry or moist soil, etc.) and he will also pitch in and help when I need him. I enjoy the time spent in the fresh air and a sense of satisfaction and accomplishment when areas of the garden are restored to their former order and beauty.

Although Russ generally has a very positive attitude coping with Parkinson's, like anyone dealing with a chronic disease, he has days when he is not feeling as fit or energetic. Some days, it's just hard to get started. Maybe he had a bad night's sleep or pushed too hard the day before. He may just be displeased or frustrated with his progress. I've learned to accept those times without judgement and let him be. Everyone needs some time alone to deal with life's ups and downs. I don't take it personally. I offer help but try to provide it only when he solicits it. I feel it's important to give him the independence he strives for.

However, sometimes a caregiver might find it necessary to give some unsolicited advice. For example, I try to let him know that sometimes he needs to slow down a bit and think about himself. Russ is a very caring and giving person. It's hard for him to put himself first. But sometimes, that has become necessary. He needs to set aside time every day for his own exercise schedule in order to feel better. As a personal trainer specializing in training people with Parkinson's, he finds it difficult to prioritize his own needs. He wants to help as many people as possible by sharing all the knowledge he has gained during his own journey. I feel it's part of my responsibility to let him know when he needs to take a break and concentrate on his own needs. Along the same lines, we need to be better about voicing his needs to others. This is something we're still working on. It can sometimes be difficult when meeting up with or having dinner with friends to coordinate the timing, so meals don't interfere with his med schedule. It's important to let them know what might be more convenient for you – true friends will always understand.

The last area I'd like to address in being a caregiver to someone with Parkinson's is support for their dietary restrictions. We've gone through many iterations from going gluten and dairy free to being totally vegan to adding back small quantities of some items like fish. Revamping our dinner menus and searching for new recipes which I think he might enjoy takes a lot of time and effort. Things are getting easier but there are still some nights when I'm frustrated with preparing dinner. Preparing vegan recipes can be labor intensive and time consuming. Keeping our scheduled dinner time in line with Russ' med schedule is another challenge. Eating too close to his med time decreases its effectiveness quite a bit so we try to keep the two schedules in sync which can lead to issues if dinner is delayed for some reason. These are all things that need to be considered as part of our daily routine.

After four years of dealing with Parkinson's Disease, Russ is still primarily independent. He is motivated to stay mentally, physically, and socially active. He has a strong desire to share his knowledge and enthusiasm with others in order to help them live the best possible life. This has made my role as his caregiver primarily supportive for the time being - listening to any new ideas and helping him to evaluate the possible advantages and disadvantages of each, giving feedback on his daily activities, being there if he needs a hand, providing the freedom for him to follow his passions and indulge in his daily routine. I am also trying to keep in mind that every caregiver needs to find some time to claim as their own. It's important for both their own health and the health of their partner.

In the future, my role as caregiver may need to become more active. But for now, our goal is to enjoy our life together and to live each day to the fullest. Although we've been somewhat stymied now by the Covid crisis, we are looking forward to getting back to attending dance socials with our friends, doing some traveling again or just going for a hike in a local park.

I've now experienced being a caregiver at both ends of the spectrum. The first experience had its challenges which were exacerbated by our lack of knowledge. From my experiences, I would encourage anyone who is diagnosed with a chronic disease to research it extensively and try to incorporate different proven treatment options into your daily routine. These might include dietary changes, addition of or modification to your exercise routine, or new drugs or supplements; but they should all be based on sound scientific research. Ask questions. Network with others dealing with the same disease. If the patient isn't up to it, this will often fall on the primary caregiver who may also be overwhelmed and may need assistance from a relative or friend. But, from my experience, the time spent is well worth it.

I don't know how much of this would have helped my mom experience a better quality of life because she didn't have the same motivation as Russ. But something as easy as changing her meal and medication schedule, asking the doctor to up the dosage of her medication or making changes to her diet may have made a difference. We'll never know. It might have made her later years more comfortable.

In any case, I know that Russ will continue to fight this disease with a passion. And when he needs me, I'll be standing in the wings ready to do whatever is necessary to keep him vibrant and vital.

Words from PD Fighter, Mike Mitani

My name is Mike Mitani, and I was diagnosed with Parkinson's in 2006 at age 56. A graduate of the US Naval Academy, my 42-year career included service in the Navy, the US Intelligence Community and overseeing advanced research projects at a large technology development company.

Pre-Diagnosis

Like many of my PD brothers and sisters, the start of my Parkinson's journey was quite unremarkable with the occasional flutter of my right foot whenever I depressed the brake pedal of my car. It was just an annoyance at the time.

I reported the symptom to the family doctor who referred me to a neurologist to rule out the possibility of something serious. After 2 visits to the specialist and a battery of tests, he rendered his opinion. "I think you have Parkinson's," he said. It was direct, clear, and unequivocal. In total shock and disbelief, I asked, "Isn't that a pretty serious diagnosis doctor?" "It could be" was his response. I spent the next 4 months seeking an alternate opinion. None came and the diagnosis stuck.

Post-Diagnosis

And so, began my Parkinson's journey of 14 years to date. A journey made infinitely more doable with the support, understanding, partnership and love of my wife of 23 years, Emily. In hindsight, I was probably showing signs at least 10 years before my official diagnosis (diminished sense of smell, disturbed sleep, and others). Over time the little flutter in my foot developed into an overall slowness of movement, rigidity, loss of dexterity, fatigue, and balance problems. Despite these challenges I feel lucky. My disease has progressed slowly, and I am functional most of the time. I take moderate doses of carbidopa/levodopa which has been prescribed to me from early on to mitigate symptoms.

As in life, there are good days and bad days with PD. Parkinson's is referred to as the great subtractive disease for a reason. PD can take away parts of your life little by little. This reality hits home every time I see my guitars and saxophone sitting idle, collecting dust in the study. Impaired dexterity and rigidity are now at a point where I can no longer play my instruments. PD can taketh away.

At the same time, I have discovered it is possible to fight back against Parkinson's – that we do not have to accept what is happening to us lying down. Beyond medications there are things we can do to change the course of the disease in our favor. I will tell you about my personal experience in this regard.

Finding Rock Steady Boxing

In November 2015 I learned of a program designed to counter or slow down the effects of PD through high intensity forced exercise, coupled with movement techniques used to train boxers in a non-contact format. With a "what do I have to lose?" attitude I joined the Rock Steady Boxing program through their local affiliate in Sacramento, Ca. Some five years later what do you know, I am still there fighting back against Parkinson's. Rock Steady has given me the training and skills necessary to wage my battle. I am convinced it has helped slow down the relentless advance of my disease.

Beyond the physical benefits, Rock Steady has given me a psychological uplift, being in a supportive environment of like-minded people sharing a common goal. The camaraderie within the fight family is readily apparent and serves as an antidote for the apathy, depression and sense of isolation that can accompany PD. Each week I look forward to having lunch with my fellow boxers after class. We have become good friends and these lunches are now a social ritual for us. This is but one of a dozen examples I could cite where the strong bonds within our fight group promote staying socially engaged and active.

Giving Back

For as long as I can recall, the notion of service has been a motivating factor in my life. The idea of thinking beyond oneself undoubtedly came from my dad who instilled in me the notion of giving back to that from which you take. In pursuit of that goal, I began contemplating ways in which I could give back to Rock Steady. As if by design, the door to an opportunity opened.

My Rock Steady Head Coach Melissa announced that she was starting up a new class for 12 additional Parkinson's boxers. It did not take long for me to ask if she could use a volunteer assistant (me) to help bring the new class into the fold. At that point I had a year of boxing under my belt and my coaching experience was connected to a totally different sport -- skiing. No matter, Melissa took a flyer on me and the rest as they say is history. The assimilation of the new class went remarkably well, and Melissa and I ended up making a great coaching tandem (in my opinion). It was gratifying to have students come up to me and tell me that my help made a difference. Little did they know that what I got back in return from them far exceeded anything I could have given them. In 2018 I successfully completed the training process to become a certified Rock Steady Boxing coach.

The Most Remarkable Individual

I will end my story with a special shout out to my Head Coach at Rock Steady Sacramento, Melissa Tafoya, without whom none of what I described above would be possible. Coach Melissa is one of the most remarkable individuals I have ever met. She teaches and motivates through her own unique blend of technical skill, imagination passion, compassion, humor and when necessary, tough love. She cares and is committed to her fighters beyond measure whether inside or outside the gym. She relentlessly encourages us to keep going when we want to stop and we respond, knowing you get out what you put in. And in the end, what you get out may be nothing less than a better quality of life with Parkinson's.

Words from Melissa Tafoya

Owner & Head Coach, Rock Steady Boxing Sacramento

Owner & Private Fitness Trainer, Multi Dimensional Training

Growing up I always felt different. I was very quiet and terrified of strangers. I was labelled 'shy' which was assumed because I was so much smaller than everyone else. I struggled in school. My Mom and I would spend hours on my homework in elementary school just to keep up. I found my voice on the playground. Tetherball was my game. As a child of the 80's, I received the reputation as the Mini Mike Tyson of tetherball.

Because of this struggle, I grew to be a voice for others who were too shy or misunderstood. I learned I had to work twice as hard as everyone else to get where I needed to be. I used this work ethic to graduate from college and nearly a decade later, put my love for hitting things and defending others together.

I became a personal trainer by happenstance. My Mom was preparing for back surgery and needed to strengthen her core. I began working out with her at the gym and was often mistaken for her trainer. In fact, the gym manager offered me a position as a personal trainer and that's how I got my start. It was clear that I loved working with people I truly care about, specifically older generations, who I am most comfortable around.

My specialty became thinking outside of the box by using a blend of unconventional training methods/strategies and compassion to help my clients regain hope and quality of life. I was constantly referred gym members with physical and neurological disorders. Often my clients were not being heard by their doctors or family members when trying to explain that something just wasn't right.

One client's neurologist was convinced she had resting tremor for two years. I questioned if it was in fact Parkinson's. I know what it's like to be misunderstood. I explained to my client that for the last several years I had been boxing and training at an amateur level which revealed my darkest demons — my social awkwardness and learning disabilities from childhood. I researched and discovered that I am Autistic. I fit the symptoms to a T. After sharing this personal story, my client would soon be diagnosed with Parkinson's.

While discovering this neurological disorder, I also discovered Rock Steady Boxing – non-contact boxing and group exercise for people with Parkinson's. I learned about the parallels between Parkinson's and Autism Spectrum Disorder. Our brains our wired differently than others – impulses, obsessive behavior, anxiety, depression, social awkwardness, learning impairments, speech, even tremor in the form of stimming. I felt equipped with my life experience to help folks just entering this chapter in their lives.

While attending a corrective exercise seminar I met a RSB coach from San Francisco, just 1-1/2 hours away from Sacramento. I became obsessed with learning more about this worldwide affiliate program. I volunteered on the weekends and fell in love with the fighters and the San Francisco program. It was time for Sacramento to have its own fight family. In 2015 I completed the training camp on my birthday and Rock Steady Boxing Sacramento was born.

Our fight family grew fast. Just two weeks after our Sacramento program launched a story on CBS Sunday Morning about the NYC affiliate aired. The most fearless people began signing up bearing so much hope and determination. They didn't know me from Adam but were didn't know what was happening to me. By this time, I had my two children, I was working and had very little social life. They also noticed my writing was in small letters and difficult to read. .

So, in 2005 I went for the first time to a Neurologist. I was them 32 years old. He told me not to worry, it was essential tremor, and he prescribed a treatment. Some years passed by and in 2011, I visited him again and he told me that he observed rigidity and more tremor. He referred me to another doctor because he thought it may be Parkinson's.

It really scared me, and I didn't do anything about it.

In 2013, I decided to go to the doctor and see what was happening. My sister and her husband are also doctors and encouraged me to see a Neurologist, Dr. Martin Mireles. He specialized in Parkinson's and irregular movements, and he was the only one in the city who did this.

As he saw me enter his office, he told me "You have Parkinson," and I just said "WHAT?"

He checked me and performed some physical tests and explained about his diagnosis. I felt sad and depressed, I wasn't able to do the simple exercises, so he prescribed me some pills and asked me to come back in a few days to see how I felt.

The medication made me feel better and upon my return to see him, he confirmed I had Parkinson's Disease. So, he explained and prescribed my treatment and told me I had to change my habits and lifestyle to try to get better.

The word PARKINSON'S really caused an impact on me, but now I just consider it only as a name to a disease. It is not who I am. And that's what I work on every day.

PD PROGRESSION

Words from PD fighter, Laura Olmos

LIVING WITH PARKINSON'S

I am Laura Olmos and I feel very happy to share my testimony as a Parkinson's Disease Fighter. I am hoping it will help other people with PD to get a better understanding of what this is all about.

My life before noticing any symptom of PD as I remember was normal and in a happy environment. My parents are both doctors (family doctor and anesthesiologist) and I have 3 sisters. I have a degree in Business Administration here in Mexico and also have a master's degree in Business Administration from Texas A & M International University, proudly with a 4.0 GPA.

Some of my out of school activities were dance classes, guitar class, swimming, and as time passed, I also took Zumba and spinning.

I had several jobs as a Comptroller in the local government, most of them having to do with Financial and Budget information. It was very demanding, but I loved my job and sometimes miss it. I reported directly to the City Mayor. I also worked with private companies doing similar activities.

EARLY SYMPTOMS - WHAT TO DO?

People around me started to ask me, why is your hand shaking, why do you walk like that, do you feel ok? I really didn't pay much of attention, until one time in a spinning class my left leg hurt. My husband also noticed some changes in me like the tremor in my hand and I walked slower. I also gained some weight because of my lack of exercise. I felt really bad about all of this and willing to take a chance. They didn't comprehend how I understood the fight, but they soon would.

Fighter after fighter continue to tell me, "I used to be somebody." Many just starting the program are intimidated and believe they are not ready. They usually explain all of their life's past achievements, as though the person who stands before me is some sort of failure. I am often told, "I'm going to get in better shape for a month or so and then start." What I explain to them so candidly is that they are ready exactly where they are. This is a group they qualify for from the get-go, and we understand. I emphasize that they should be proud of the fighter they are choosing to become and the family they have joined.

The biggest symptom and the most common I see in my Champs is a symptom from society. They are waiting for the perfect time to start. The apathy is also great, but this idealism of where they are supposed to be is so strong that they waste precious time. Most are already diagnosed at least 10 years after first exhibiting symptoms. I explain that each moment matters. Each day matters. Waiting for the perfect opportunity exacerbates the problem.

When the 2020 Pandemic hit, we sheltered inside immediately. Structure and routine is imperative for people on the spectrum and people with Parkinson's. Our Champs learned to adapt to Zoom Happy Hours to socialize weekly, virtual workouts on Facebook Live and later Zoom. They were held accountable to the same weekly workout schedule that now included supply lists sent daily of household equipment they would need to use during their workouts: paper plates, broomsticks, soup cans, a chair, etc. By this time, most of our Champs had been in our fight family for a minimum of six months, many for four plus years. They had overcome their fear of technology and jumped right in knowing they were not alone.

As the Pandemic's intensity increased and our programed

remained remote, our Champs began reaching out to one another, even scheduling meet ups and bike rides at distance. They stopped waiting for our return to the gym and found ways of making connections. It has been my experience that people with Parkinson's are the most exceptional people. They have the unwavering ability to find purpose and fight for something greater than themselves, the quality of life for each other.

As the saying goes, if you've met one person with Parkinson's, you've met one person with Parkinson's. The diversity of symptoms and personalities in our fight fam was brilliant, but the diversity of race was absent. This held true attending annual Parkinson's conferences, workshops, and support groups in the greater Sacramento area. This lack of diversity was like the white elephant in the room. This troubled me for years, but I did nothing.

Seeing this disparity, I asked myself, how can I stand up for individual people I care about, but not an entire population? It was obvious that a whole demographic was being overlooked, people of color with Parkinson's. I made excuses of why I couldn't get involved. I too was wasting precious time. I certainly don't take excuses from my fighters, why was I exempt? With the recent murder of George Floyd and the uprising of our current civil rights movement, I no longer felt restrained to say nothing out of fear of what to do. The time is now. This inner call to action led me to start a grass roots endeavor: Health Disparities and Parkinson's in Sacramento, Ca.

We are forming concentric circles of advocacy. I consider this an extension of my fight family. My team consists of three women:

1. Denise Coley: Black advocate and woman living with Parkinson's

2. Gena Lennon: Parkinson's Foundation Development Manager-Sacramento & Fresno

3. Melissa Tafoya: Latinx advocate and fitness coach for people with Parkinson's

We are having warm Zoom calls in order to start organic conversations with people of color in our community. We are listening and learning about what barriers are preventing this engagement. We are doing the fieldwork to collect this key information and share resources from the Parkinson's Foundation. Our goal is to develop access, make connections for engagement to resources for the improved quality of life and hope for people with Parkinson's in Sacramento.

Never in my life have I felt so much love and so much purpose. I wake up every day excited to see my Champs and private clients, or as I often call them, my kids. Whether it be via Zoom, park workouts, an email, or phone-call during our state shutdown, these connections feed my soul. Having peers and friends like Karl Sterling, only enrich my life that much further. Not a day goes by that I'm not reading an article, participating in a webinar, or reading a new book about neuroscience and health disparities in Parkinson's. I can't stop feeding my mind and my heart. I remain eternally grateful for this Parkinson's community.

Words from PRT Instructor, Luis Rubén Artavia

I slept &dreamed that life is all joy.
I woke & saw that life is all service.
I served & saw that service is joy.
- Kahlil Gibran

"I'll see you at the bar." This was Karl's invitation to connect and the beginning of a game changer journey for me.

I was born and raised in San José, Costa Rica. Blessed with the most supportive family that taught me about love and tolerance as fundamental values to whatever I wanted to accomplish in life.

I never believed in coincidences and that's why meeting Karl felt positive and powerful since the beginning. His authentic, unselfish way to communicate opened my mind and heart to learn what has become my real path to follow.

His program started by having his first PD client without asking for it. Traveling around the world, asking questions, and humbly listening to what others have to say gave the Parkinson's Regeneration Training a real identity in this amazing industry.

Understanding their different conditions, having tools to improve their physical and cognitive state, and caring about people around you; are just a few of the highlights of Karl's program.

As a fitness trainer this is a whole new way for me to impact someone else's quality of life. "Real results," I used to say when we started helping people roll out of bed in the morning, trained them for functional independence and improving their family and social environment in general.

Treating the person in front of you as a whole system, physically, mentally, emotionally, and spiritually has become the most important assessment to contribute.

We don't care anymore about the condition or the disease's name. WHO is the person you want to help? What does he/she like to do? How can we help them smile more and live another day for their loved ones?

This exciting new professional experience and view of life has impacted my personal way of living, too.

Listening to patients around the world, paying attention to what they have to say, how they feel, how they live and my calling to positively impact others has reminded me that love is still the answer for everything.

"This is not Karl's show." "This is not even the PRT show." Both Karl's statements that always lead to other professionals to contribute to the table and create a massive environment of good intentions and causalities everywhere we engage.

It's not all perfect. Working close to people with little or no hope can bring us down and weaken our system instead. The biggest challenge is to keep yourself together and be willing to share energy and time with whoever needs it the most.

A dynamic balance between being vulnerable and consciously listening to what life needs from you, is the real deal. We are just human beings surviving to nature, we forgot about that a long time ago. Is there a way to remember our roots as social creatures?

This has been my biggest surprise. Understanding the great influence that people around us have in the way we perceive life. Not to blame our environment or values but to appreciate them to overcome whatever life brings tomorrow.

My purpose wasn't clear; I didn't know where I was going or why I was doing it. It was just one of those strong gut feelings that took me to the bar with Karl.

We all have a purpose in life and our only goal should be, to be ready for when it comes.

Three years later my life has changed, my perception of stress and pain has shifted. Now I understand that life is not about looking for happiness but to choose with our hearts what are we going to be not happy about.

Parkinson's, Alzheimer's, brain paralysis and other chronic diseases out there must be treated individually for what the person really needs to live fully and enjoy their days, not just as a medical name that defines them.

Depression, anxiety, and other emotional crisis are here, and it is our job as a society to raise awareness and help everyone the universe puts in our path.

Sometimes it feels like "coincidence," and sometimes we do plan for it. At the end of the day, it is about being aware and open to it.

We have contributed to all different human beings around the world. We have shared their sadness and joy. We've talked, eaten, and danced together. The most beautiful thing though, is realizing that THEY have healed US instead.

It doesn't even matter who you are, what's your major or where you came from; knock on your neighbor's door and offer your service. We are here to be inspired by all the practices of life and to inspire whoever needs our good energy, too.

Words from PRT Instructor, Alison Klaum

Through my work as a personal trainer based in western Massachusetts and my travels as an instructor for Parkinson's Regeneration Training, I have had the honor of training and becoming a part of the lives of many people with Parkinson's (PwP) in different parts of the country.

This story, however, begins with those PwP I could not reach, those I could not help. I begin with their stories because even though I could not help them directly using the tools I have learned about movement and the brain in my years working in the fitness industry, these individuals have significantly shaped the focus of my career. They are the reason that I work with those with PD and other movement disorders. And their stories are a reminder that sometimes the greatest influences in our lives are borne out of failures and loss, and the greatest connections, from other disconnections, or connections we fail to make.

Years before I entered the fitness industry, my grandfather was diagnosed with PD. I watched along with the rest of my family as he struggled with the difficult side effects of Parkinson's, many of which I did not really understand at the time. Watching him struggle to move his legs when he tried to walk and his inability to steady his hand enough to feed himself a cupcake I brought him for his 88th birthday still haunt me. While these experiences were unsettling, they taught me invaluable lessons. They granted me personal insight into the feelings of helplessness loved ones and caregivers of those with PD can endure. In turn, through my work as a fitness professional, this insight has helped me to empower those caring for PwP by arming them with movement and "brain training" techniques for their loved ones. And while it still stings to know that I may have been able to help my grandfather navigate the challenges of PD if I knew then what I know now, I am reassured that he helped set me on the path to helping others with this disease.

Another important influence in my career path was my former mother-in-law, who, years after I lost my grandfather, was also diagnosed with PD. At the time of her diagnosis, I had recently changed careers and begun working in the fitness industry. It was also around this time that I saw Karl Sterling's post on social media about his Parkinson Regeneration Training, a movement and brain-based program designed to help fitness trainers work with PwP and caregivers. Though I had met Sterling earlier that year at a fitness event in NYC, I knew nothing of his program until I saw that fateful post on Facebook. And had it not been for my mother-in-law's (MiL) recent diagnosis, which had brought PD back to the forefront of my thoughts, I would have overlooked it. The timing of everything seemed perfect. Realizing I could focus my career on working with those with movement disorders, as well as finding a way of honoring my grandfather's memory and a way of being of service to my MiL, was a revelation. PRT helped to open up another world of possibility—one in which my personal and professional life intertwined in a meaningful and unexpected way.

Yet all of this apparent serendipity was bittersweet. A subsequent divorce later that same year and many thousands of physical miles separating me from my MiL ultimately prevented me from working with her directly. Knowing that she is fighting the disease on the other side of the world beyond my reach deeply saddens me to this day. This missed connection, however, not only led me to find PRT but also has driven me to help others in ways that I have been unable to help her.

Sterling's PRT program introduced me to several larger categories and templates of movement that still form the basis of my client sessions. They include "primal" floor-based movements, coordination/balance exercises, and cognitive/movement challenges. Because not every client responds well to the same specific exercise, trainers need to be problem-solvers and having a series of templates as well as an understanding of a movement concept helps me to be creative when designing programs tailored to my clients' specific needs. Ultimately, the application of these broader movement categories during individual client sessions has led to stronger, more resilient clients who are better prepared to resist falls and overcome the struggles they encounter on a daily basis.

Aside from specific movement-based approaches, PRT introduced me to the importance of engendering a sense of fun and encouraging play during client sessions. While this seemed to happen naturally during our weekend long PRT workshops, it proved more challenging when I tried to re-create it in my individual client sessions. This difficulty stemmed in part from my own personal hang-ups when I was still trying to figure out who I was as a trainer early in my career. I was eager to demonstrate my professionalism and my serious approach to a serious disease: I was "all business" when it came to PD and to client sessions. My motivation may have been earnest/genuine, but the sessions were flat, uninspiring.

Ultimately it was my PwP clients that truly taught me to loosen up and accept that taking something seriously—especially taking myself seriously—does not necessitate rejecting playfulness and laughter. In fact, I discovered that my "seriousness"—or, really, uptightness—was preventing me from making deeper, more meaningful connections to my clients. They helped me see that curiosity, a sense of play/fun, and a sense of humor can not only lead to more successful training sessions, but also help someone cope with the disease and the struggles of life in general. This invaluable lesson has transformed me as a trainer—and as a person.

These qualities—fun, humor, play, and curiosity—now form the cornerstone of my client sessions; they are just as important as the selection of exercises. These elements are organically shaped by a client's personality, individual needs, and the trust and rapport I build with each one of them. As a result, the ways in which these qualities manifest during a session varies from client to client, and even from session to session. In some cases, it might involve an hour of me and my client playfully ribbing each other while I lead them through their exercise routine. For others, it might mean gamifying the challenge of getting on and off the floor. For still others, it might involve letting off steam (and building hand-eye coordination!) by batting a balloon around for part of a session.

Without a doubt, working with PwP and other movement disorders has been the most gratifying part of my life. And now more than ever our connections and the work we do together has become even more significant during these times of uncertainty and increased isolation. From my grandfather and my former MiL who first inspired me to learn more about PD, from Karl Sterling's transformative approach to working with PwP, and from the indomitable spirit of the clients with whom I work every week, I have learned so much and am forever indebted. I truly believe I have the best job in the world.

Words from José Eleuterio González Martínez M.D.

I began to see patients with Parkinson's disease when I was studying Sports Medicine and Rehabilitation in the city of Monterrey, Nuevo León, Mexico. Working with Parkinson's patients leaves you a lot of life lessons, since patients see life in a different way, they enjoy the day to day, they bond more with their families and they become better people, in addition they fight to improve their quality of life whatever the cost (physically speaking). It is something that inspires us as doctors to see life differently and leaves us learning. And the truth is that Parkinson's in books is one thing and in real life it's another. Not only do you have to work the physical, but also the emotional. I remember on one occasion, a very young patient of around 48 years old, who was recently diagnosed with Parkinson's, told me that she was very sad because she felt useless and no longer felt like a woman. Most patients when told that they have Parkinson's disease go into some depression, even if it is mild or not very noticeable Parkinson's, they still feel sad, and that is where the first challenge begins.

One of the things that we tell patients is that, if we carry out a good rehabilitation, the patient will have a good quality of life, since together with the medicine and therapeutic exercise the patient will gradually improve. Something very important that I comment to my patients is that the treatment is multidisciplinary: neurologist, psychiatrist / psychologist, geriatrician, rehabilitator and the most important of all… the family.

The latter, the family, plays an important role in the management of this disease, since with them we support ourselves so that the patient feels better, gains strength, but, above all, that they support us so that the patient does not give up. It is incredible how the family gives such great support that, by itself, it provides 50% of the patient's improvement. On another occasion, a 55-year-old female patient, diagnosed with Parkinson's, told me how her husband, who used to be a person who spent his time and money on alcohol, gave up all his vice to take care of his wife. I remember that they commented that those last years, despite the illness, had been the best years of their lives. The patient continues with her rehabilitation program and is physically independent.

On another occasion, another patient, a 60-year-old male, several years after the diagnosis, began to see life differently and began to share his way of thinking with people, to the extent that he started a new business giving lectures motivational for people.

One of the main causes of death in patients with Parkinson's disease is medical complications derived from fractures, due to falls. And this is a very important topic because it is a fundamental part of the rehabilitation program: prevention of falls.

In addition, something fundamental that we must work with patients is the speed of the gait, since it is a predictor of mortality, thus, if a patient takes more than 5 seconds to walk 4 meters, the mortality at one year is 60%. And if we improve our walking and speed, mortality decreases.

In rehabilitation there are different objectives: to improve gait, mobility, coordination, balance, flexibility, breathing exercises, trunk control and cognitive rehabilitation. To work on all these objectives, we must do it little by little, so as not to fatigue the patient, since fatigue is one of the causes of attrition of patients. Also, the exercises should be fun, entertaining and vary the exercises session by session.

The routine that we do with patients is 3 times a week, in which we include aerobic exercise with a stationary bike, strengthening with rubber bands and medicine ball, in addition, we work strength with vibration exercises with a vibrating platform, also balance exercises and proprioception with rockers and stabilizers, gait re-education with parallel bars, and when the patient has improved his gait, we begin to work gait coordination with a floor ladder and cones. We perform trunk control with exercises with a yoga ball and breathing exercises with an inspirometer. We also perform multitasking exercises for cognitive rehabilitation, and we always do physical therapy, to maintain joint mobility and muscle stretching exercises.

One of the most difficult obstacles is that patients drop out of rehabilitation programs, because improvement is slow and rehabilitation programs may not have an end. Sometimes the patient is very willing to finish his program, but as in many cases, the patients are older adults, they do not have the way to move by themselves and they depend on their children to bring them to their therapy. On many occasions, this is one of the reasons why patients do not finish their program. That is when we as doctors enter into talking with the children and trying to convey the importance of the rehabilitation program, that the objectives are important and that little by little the patient will improve. It is not easy to work all the points in patients with Parkinson's, since different challenges are presented along the way that must be overcome. Each patient experiences the disease in different ways, some fall into a total depression, others find a better way to live life and others take advantage and even hold conferences to help people. We must support the patient physically and emotionally.

Personally, Parkinson's disease has taught me a lot, seeing how patients look for all possible ways to get ahead, it is a true example of life, in addition, we see how during their therapeutic exercise, although physically they can no longer, they seek by doing an extra repetition, one more series, they seek to improve each session, do the exercises better than the previous session, and not only improve in their exercise sessions, they also continue with their rehabilitation at home.

But the most emotional of all is to see how the patient achieves his independence and how he maintains himself over time, and to always keep going.

To you, as a doctor, I tell you that you must always look ahead, and that no matter how many difficulties you have along the way, if you keep fighting, following medical indications, undoubtedly your life will be very independent, and Parkinson's will go into the background. Live in the moment, join your family more and sooner rather than later, you will see great results. José Eleuterio González Martínez M.D.

Sports Medicine and Rehabilitation

Words from Dr. Eduardo Guadarrama Molina

My name is Eduardo Guadarrama Molina, I am a 31-year-old doctor living in the city of Monterrey, Mexico for 6 years now. I specialize in Sports Medicine and Rehabilitation. The athlete is one of the patients we examine in this specialty for injuries, preventive measures, and evaluations of their performance. Also, at the University I attended, we saw patients who needed rehabilitation related to other medical services, such as rheumatology, plastic surgery, endocrinology, cardiology, traumatology, and neurology. In neurology, I met Dr. Ingrid Estrada Bellmann, a neurologist specializing in Parkinson's disease and abnormal movements. She suggested that I do a research study where neurology and sports medicine and rehabilitation work together, which I could use as a degree thesis. We organized and decided to work with Parkinson's disease patients evaluating a rehabilitation modality.

Throughout the study, I met many patients with this disease. They had a first evaluation to meet us, the medical history, the balance test and explain what their rehabilitation would consist of. I was well accepted by the patients, as they began to notice clinical improvement and that made them happy and motivated. At the final evaluation, it was very satisfying to see the patient with a different countenance, with enthusiasm, with energy, with more movement and less rigidity. It was motivating for me to observe the great changes that were seen on exploration, and likewise, the emotion that was highlighted in them. Dr. Ingrid would see the patients after the end of the study,

enthusiastically telling me about the changes that the patients exhibited. This is where we find the true importance of rehabilitation and exercise in patients with Parkinson's disease not only in their clinical condition, also in their psychological condition, improving their mood, their enthusiasm, and their motivation. As a result, I had great pleasure in working with these patients.

Although we know that it is a disease that has no cure and is a degenerative disease, the improvement depends a lot on each patient, being at times frustrating when observing that the clinical changes they can become slightly visible or almost nonexistent. This also leads me to tell each patient that patience is an important tool, dedication and perseverance are valuable to find significant improvement, that they do not fall into despair and working hard they will be able to return to their previous quality of life.

From all this experience, I participated in various activities related to Parkinson's disease, such as conferences, talks to patients, participation in Congresses talking about the importance of rehabilitation, activation sessions for patients and meeting many people who also share that affection for helping people with this condition.

During my specialty I met many patients. I remember one of them with a moderate degree of the disease, he went to the rehabilitation department for sessions on a device called an oscillating bed. The patient arrived with a bit of freezing of gait, with difficulty in articulating words, and after 20 minutes of his session the symptoms decreased significantly. He went to his therapy session twice a week. I spoke with him and told him about the study we were conducting, but he was not a candidate for it. There came a time when the device had failures, so he could not take his therapy. For this reason, the patient had a relapse, accentuating the symptoms. He sought me out and we organized a therapeutic training plan and returning to improvement.

There was another patient who also sought me out through Dr. Ingrid who has more pronounced and severe symptoms (with gait problems). We began his rehabilitation and there was slight improvement. The disease was already well established. One day he arrived with a laser stick, which emitted a strip on the ground to help him as a visual aid in the gait. This laser stick did not help him much and we did a test with a conventional stick, and we put a plastic strap in the lower part about 3-5 cm high, helping the patient more as a visual aid. One time, instead of arriving in a wheelchair driven by his caregiver, he arrived by motorized car, and he began to miss rehabilitation therapies and left exercising at home, neglecting himself a lot and therefore relapsed and accentuated the symptoms.

These two cases mentioned above help to understand the importance of rehabilitation and exercise in this disease. Both cases, having good control, follow-up, and adherence, had excellent results, however, by setting aside consistency and abandoning physical therapy, they showed a regression and worsening of the disease. In the same way, technological and modern aids have taken a great step forward in humanity and in Parkinson's disease by saving us the effort in something so beneficial and free that we have within our reach, and that is exercise. There are countless ways to activate and exercise, there are many ways to improvise utensils that can help us in exercise therapy, making it clear that the most sophisticated, new, or luxurious device is not necessary to obtain the benefits of exercise and physical activation.

Words from Ted Byrd: Misdiagnosed with Parkinson's

My name is Ted Byrd, and I was diagnosed with Parkinson's on February 2, 2021. I am a husband, a father, a grandfather (known as "Boppi" to my grandkids), a Navy veteran, a teacher of 20 years, a former mechanic, born and raised in Syracuse, NY. My Interests include reading, watching football, comic books, and teaching. I just retired this year due to the symptoms I was experiencing.

My journey began in August of 2019 when I went to the VA for a completely different reason. I had a crush injury to my right hand, which had to be re-evaluated due to it getting worse. I was sent to see a VA neurologist, who at that time diagnosed me with PD. I was in complete shock and disbelief because I had no symptoms that aligned with Parkinson's.

In August 2020 I fell in my garage, bruising my tailbone. Not long after that, I started stumbling periodically while walking. After struggling for months and realizing that I definitely had something wrong with my right leg, I knew I needed to seek medical attention. In January of 2021, I went to see a neurosurgeon. My right calf had severe pain, my toes would go up, not curl under, and I would walk on the ball of my foot. This would often cause me to lunge for things to keep me upright, which sometimes didn't work, and down on the floor I went… Thank God I didn't get hurt. Getting back to the appointment, the doctor sent me for MRIs of the back and brain...he found nothing (go ahead, laugh). And the adventure continues… He referred me to a neurologist. My wife, formerly a nurse in a neurology office, got me an appointment with the head neurologist. At my appointment he did a neurological exam. He concluded that I have PD, prescribed carbidopa/levodopa, and just said "I'll see you in 6 months." I thought: "What the hell just happened?"

I was devastated. I had just been handed a life sentence of PD. As everyone knows, there are different stages. I was in denial. It had such a profound impact on my family and relationships. It also affected me mentally, I was depressed, and could not see a light at the end of the tunnel.

We then asked for a referral to see a Movement Disorder Specialist in Rochester, NY. This is where, I was told, the best in the area are doing their practice. The doctor made the referral but said the diagnosis would be the same. The office of the MDS called and said that it would not be for another 4 months before she could see me!

Due to me not being able to move well, I felt I had to leave work before I was ready to retire, especially since I worked in a jail. Obviously, the doctor was not going to do anything but give me medication, which did nothing. I had to do things for myself. I felt it was up to me to "to take the bull by the horns," so to say. I joined groups online and did research; Learned everything through my own search for answers. I searched for physical therapists and that is when I met Liz and started LSVT-BIG. Everything was going great...that is until my leg/foot wouldn't work correctly. The symptoms that I researched did not line up with what my body was doing. However, I have also learned that everyone does not have the same symptoms when it comes to PD which is what makes it so damn hard to diagnose and find a cure!

In my search for answers, I went on Amazon and found a book titled "Parkinson's Regeneration Training" authored by Karl Sterling. I ordered the book and started to read it. To my surprise, I found out that Karl Sterling is from Syracuse, NY as well and works locally! Taking a chance, I googled to see if I could find Karl's phone number. I called the number and was surprised when Karl actually answered the phone to an unknown number (a thing he has admitted to me that he often does not do). I proceeded to tell him what I was going through and asked if he could help me. I was surprised by his answer: "Yes, I believe I can." This was the start of a beautiful friendship.

Every time I would go in to see Karl, he would say "Let's try X. It's an experiment!" I could see the wheels turning. Then Karl would say "Well that didn't work. Let's try something else!" I have learned so much from Karl, but the most important thing is to never give up. I could end here but please bear with me just a little while longer. The most important part of my story hasn't been told yet.

Everyone where my wife worked (a doctor's office) asked If I had had a nerve conduction study done. This test should have been one of the first tests given to me. Months later, they did give me an EMG, from which they found pinched nerves at the S1-L5. I asked the doctor who did the EMG if that could be the cause of my problems that they had previously blamed on Parkinson's: the pain in the calf, the toes going up in the air, taking short steps, weakness, and the leg trying to buckle. "Yes" he said, "that could cause all of that."

Well September 10th came; it was the day of my Movement Disorder Specialist appointment (4 months in the making). I was horribly anxious and dreading it. When we arrived at the clinic, we were shown to the MDS's office. She came in and introduced herself and proceeded to ask my wife and I a series of questions. She then examined me using the typical neurological movement tests for PD. I told her about my immobility problems with my leg and so she then observed me walking using my walker. As she observed, she asked if I was in pain. I told her that yes, I was having pain in my right calf. She said she could tell due to the way I was walking. She then took me back into her office to sit down. This was the part of the appointment I was dreading: her confirmation that I do indeed have PD. This is what she said: "I see Parkinson's patients every day, all day. It is my medical opinion that you do not have Parkinson's." Almost instantaneously, it was as if a weight had been lifted off my shoulders. She said I should follow up on the pinched nerves that she saw in my file and in her medical opinion, I no longer needed to focus on PD. Despite my relief, I had mixed emotions.

Without even actually having it, Parkinson's Disease had brought me anxiety, fear, sadness, and really made me think about my life. However, it also improved my life immensely, I started exercising, ate "green stuff" and salads, and became closer with friends and family. I went to the doctor, sought out physical therapy, talked openly with people like Liz about stress and feelings, and found a sense of community.

Although I do not in fact have Parkinson's Disease, I am sharing my story in order to encourage others to be their own advocate. Push for testing, seek out help from any and all resources, and don't be afraid to get a second opinion...or a third. Maybe if they had done an EMG sooner, it would have saved me a lot of pain and frustration. To this day, I still do not have a definitive diagnosis but through this journey, I have learned to advocate for myself and will continue to do so until the doctors give me answers. You need to fight for yourself. Be your own advocate, because not everyone has Karl in their korner.

Words from trainer, Sylvie Patrick

I met Michelle in 2016 during a member's workshop that I was giving in her Country Club.

The workshop provided basic information on how to use a whole-body vibration platform to warm up and recover pre and post workout. I had done many of these workshops and always enjoy the members interaction. Most of the participants were over 60 years of age and were physically active and in apparent good health.

Michelle approached me at the end of my presentation and asked me if I have used vibrations with clients suffering from Parkinson. I did not know if she was asking for herself or someone else, I answered that I had a few clients with Parkinson taking classes in my training studio and they seemed to get better mobility and balance once they were exposed to vibrations. However, I mentioned that the class format was not designed to specifically address their needs. She promised to reach out with more questions, and we left it at this.

You need some context to understand where I was career wise when I started with Michelle.

When I opened my training studio in 2007, I had quit my corporate job and a comfortable 6 figures salary to start a new career in fitness. I decided to focus my new business on vibrations training and grabbed a niche that no one was offering.

The boutique studio concept was inexistent, and many thought I was crazy to open a 900 sq ft training studio with 7 vibration machines to offer small group classes across the street of a Gold's Gym. I had a clear business plan, and I thought my clientele would be essentially women in their 30s and 40s who needed to lose a few pounds while juggling with work and kids.

However, after a few years in business, the reality hit. My main clients were over 50 years old, needed better mobility, good balance and, although losing weight was still on their wish list, it was clear that it was not the priority for them to stay healthy and active.

I was lacking the education to deal with aging population and needed to learn and look for mentors.

This is how I got introduced to the Functional Aging Institute, Evidence Based Fitness Academy, and 3DMap from Gray Institute.

I gained experience dealing with clients who had multiple sclerosis, Parkinson's, diabetes, neuropathy, lymphedema, knee and hip replacement, osteoporosis, and lots of golf injuries. However, I had never designed a personal training program to work one on one with a client diagnosed with Parkinson's in order to improve life.... until Michelle called back.

For our first session, I planned on using the same movement assessment protocol as with the rest of my clients and I assumed her fitness goals would probably be in line with them too.

When we met the first time, I asked her how Parkinson's had affected her life since her diagnosis a couple of years ago. She had trouble sleeping, bad digestion, difficulty focusing, and stiffness in the morning causing muscle aches. She also could not write very well and was sometimes losing her balance. She did not have any tremors nor hallucinations.

She was told by her physician that being active could help her slow down the progression of the disease. She started to use the recumbent bike and elliptical in her country club fitness center a couple of days per week.

She just wanted to feel confident and reassured that she will be able to continue to enjoy life with her husband and family.

Listening to her and asking questions about her family and lifestyle via a casual conversation is my way to do my Part Q. I usually share the fact that I am from France and suddenly learned that my client used to travel, wanted to plan family vacations; revealing a level of activity that they would not have necessarily shared otherwise.

Her training program was designed to help her feel stronger and prepare her for all the projects she had.

Assessing movements was challenging from the start. It seems that she could not understand my cueing.

I modified the 3DMap assessment because she was confused and loss balance in the same side lateral moves, which involve reaching with one foot on each side of the other foot part of the supporting leg. Crossing one foot in front of the other was almost impossible for her and I could tell how dangerous it could be, gaiting with sudden change of direction, with this lack of stability and control.

I used a new client form to keep track of score and make comments. You can obtain this form on the book support website at www.thepdbook.org

Words from trainer, Lilia Drew

I began my journey as a personal trainer working in a private country club. The average age was 75. Being 25 and having recently obtained my certification as personal trainer, my first few months were to say the least, challenging!

I have always been what I consider to be a good learner. I enjoy learning new things and applying them to real life. I obtained a bachelor's degree in International Business because I was told I should. I quickly realized it wasn't my passion when I was introduced to the Fitness Industry. I did well studying Business, but I LOVED studying for my personal training certification. Seeing how muscles worked together, or opposite, to create movement was better than watching a good episode of Seinfeld. Through connections, I was very fortunate to have my first job at this pristine, private club fitness center. However, as I mentioned earlier, the average age was 75.

When you study the anatomy of the body, it seems very easy to be able to take what the book says and apply it on your clients. I quickly learned that as people age, their bodies change immensely, and there isn't one body that is similar to the other, especially the bodies in the textbook! This challenge made me further my education in exercise science, in which I realized that with the human body, you can never know enough. It is very true that the more you know, the less you know.

My first client with Parkinson's was Mr. Kauffer, referred to me by his massage therapist. I thought I knew a bit about Parkinson's disease; tremors, typically more as people aged, I was familiar with Michael J. Fox. Looking back, he was in early stages, had been active his entire life, didn't have many tremors. His main complaint was that he felt stiff, loss of balance and noticed he had trouble moving his ankles. We developed a great relationship; I thought I was

"Doing a fantastic job with him!" We completed our workouts; however, the stiffness never would go away, and my protocols of balance and mobility weren't really going anywhere. In all honesty, my workouts weren't as specific as they should have been for having Parkinson's Disease, but we continued to train together for years. Every completed workout gave him a sense of achievement and hope of regaining a bit of what 'normal' life used to be.

I was soon referred Mr. Dixon. He had never worked with a personal trainer, however had heard that exercise was beneficial. He was definitely in a later stage of Parkinson's. He had trouble sleeping, loss of balance, dizziness, tremors, extremely high and low blood pressure amongst other symptoms.

Mr. Dixon was a little more of a challenge, yet very inspirational to work with. He never missed a workout, no matter how low his energy was or how he felt. He worked his hardest in every session. He wanted so badly to 'get better, which at times caused a bit of depression.

These clients made me want to learn as much as I could about Parkinson's disease. I had worked with many clients with different ailments; however, Mr. Kauffer and Mr. Dixon were special. They gave 110% every session. They had to work harder than any other person to simply feel 'normal,' or what they remembered as being normal. They wanted so bad to feel what healthy individuals take for granted.

I shortly after studied and certified in the Parkinson's Regeneration Training. The material and seminar were phenomenal. The course truly gave me the understanding of how Parkinson's disease affects the brain, and how each modality of exercise has its purpose and importance. For example, cardiovascular activity creates Brain Derived Neurotrophic Factor, which regenerate cells in the brain, allowing for communication from brain to body, flexibility to lessen feeling of rigidity, balance, and much more. With this new knowledge and understanding, my sessions became better structured and much more fun!

I can honestly say I love working with individuals with Parkinson's. I have found them to be so determined that they work harder than other clients. They know what it is to wake up every day not feeling 100% yet remember what it felt like to feel 'normal'. Although you cannot regress symptoms of Parkinson's, you definitely can slow the Progression, which becomes the goal. Every small achievement during workouts is a huge victory, which brings confidence and joy in everyday life. The exercises that we do carry on to daily tasks

If I had to say there is some challenge in training individuals with Parkinson's disease, I would have to say patience and how to overcome frustration. I cannot imagine waking up every day not having control of my body, and slowly losing ability to do activities I enjoyed. Often some exercise that seem easy feel very challenging. But the more frustrated the client gets, the more the difficulty. It's important to step back, take a big breath, and break up the task piece by piece. Every day is a different day, which is how I treat my sessions. Every day has its own challenges and its own rewards.

I am thankful every day for what my clients teach me. Whenever I come across a struggle in my life, whether physically or mentally, I think of what they deal with every second of their lives. How they would love to be able to do the things I do. Things I don't even have to think about that is often impossible to them. Each of them has impacted me in different ways. My time with them is so rewarding and inspirational.

Words from PD fighter, Alfredo Bozziere

My name is Alfredo Bozziere Gallardo, and I am 42 years old. I am a professional, a Biologist. For 12 years, I have been teaching at a technical middle school level in the town of Rinconada, Veracruz.

I was a healthy and educated child, always worried about others, very calm and involved. I always demonstrated the characteristics of a great leader. I believe this distinguishes me from the group of people that surround me. I have been playing sports since I was nine years old. I was distinguished by my strength, skills, and abilities, and my endurance and speed.

I was a centered, committed, and hardworking person before my life with Parkinson's Disease started. I currently continue with my physical exercises of alpinism and mountain biking. I was an exemplary athlete because of my strength, intellect, speed, and performance on the mountain route. I felt like I could do anything that I set my mind to do. Even when I did not have complete knowledge of certain activities, I always tried since I wanted to be the best. I always wanted to contribute. However, there came a moment in my life where I began to feel that my body was behaving strangely. I began to develop certain movements and certain difficulties that prevented me from doing everyday activities.

One day while writing on the class blackboard, I began to feel a stiffness in my right arm as well as pain in the arm and shoulder blade area. This worried me as I could not even write anymore. My index finger slowly started to move. I went to a traumatologist, and he told me I had a problem in my spine and mentioned that vertebrae were hurting me and that is why I felt that way. Even with antibiotics, I still did not notice any improvement.

I began to feel more stiffness and movement in my right arm. Sometimes I would completely stop writing even though I did not want to. I would grab my shirt as if I were to remove it, but it was not voluntary.

I decided to consult with an internist, and he redirected me to a neurologist. He just took one glance at me and said, "You have Parkinson's Disease" to what I responded, "How am I going to have Parkinson's? I'm only 27 years old." The doctor did a CT scan to confirm it was Parkinson's to which he was right. The neurologist informed me about the surgeries and deep stimulation implants in Mexico City. His recommendation was for me to find a way to get to the Hospital General Siglo XXI.

When I got home after the doctor's appointment, I started crying. I lay down on my bed and stayed there for eight days. I was sad, depressed, and I could not believe it. How was it possible that a healthy, vice-free, 27-year-old was diagnosed with Parkinson's Disease? I only wanted to help others and was worried about my students' learning.

Even though my depression was strong, I kept going and decided to keep going forward. Getting out of bed was a pretty strong change in attitude for me. It was a reminder that I was not giving up. As it was a chronic degenerative condition, I would have to face it and live as best as I could. I decided to do something about it and not stop my usual activities, which were what got me going.

The disease continued to evolve. I began to shake with stiffness, I was depressed, and my body, although it was still working, felt different. I continued playing soccer and did my mountaineering and cycling activities. This became a personal challenge for me, and I was not leaving the sport.

The years passed and I made it to the Hospital General Siglo XXI, and my neurosurgeon gave me more information on the surgery. He explained that they would do an injury to the brain where they would introduce and retire a needle. They said this would help me improve. After the surgery, there was going to be more time to make the Deep Stimulation Implant. I agreed to have the injury done with water and the two years after that I felt much better. Unfortunately, the symptoms began to show shortly after that. I tried remedies, massages, medications, anything that would help but without favorable results.

It was only when I decided to change my attitude and accept my suffering that I went back to work to be an example and help others. My goal was to become an example for my students and the people that surround me.

Today, at 16 years of this disease's evolution, I keep moving forward, exercising, and putting a lot of effort into my bike training. I try to travel the longest distance daily and get involved in routes with more experienced people in cycling and alpinism. Without a doubt, my most difficult challenge living with Parkinson's Disease is the abandonment of some of my loved ones. They could not bear the thought of living with a person that would need a caregiver. The second most difficult challenge is depression. I am tired of not doing simple things like eating, showering, shaving, or changing by myself.

I take around 20 to 25 pills per day. I have tried many different things, but the price of medicine is very high. I worry about depression because it often comes during inappropriate moments, and it leads me to make erroneous decisions. I have a strong attitude and keep on training on the bike. I have fallen but so far, I have not hurt myself. I am still waiting for Deep Stimulation Implant surgery. I have all the studies but, due to the coronavirus, they cannot perform the surgery. I have hope and faith that one day they will do the surgery. I am 42 years old; I still have a long way to go and many people to help. I want to do what I love without problems.

Sometimes it is difficult to face this condition, but I do not give up. It is sad to know that I am going to be locked in a body. I will not be able to walk, and at an early age, I will cease to exist. I am interested in leaving a legacy, a story of overcoming, of work, of everyday training, and wanting to have a better quality of life. I am afraid of being forgotten but, I want young people to see in me a motivation to get ahead.

For me, this is Parkinson's Disease.

Bibliography

A, L. (2006, January). *Depression in Parkinson's disease -- a review.* Retrieved from US National Library of Medicine National Institutes of Health: https://www.ncbi.nlm.nih.gov/pubmed/16367891

Aaron Kucinskia, R. L. (2015, April 1). *Science Direct.* Retrieved from Behavioural Brain Research: https://www.sciencedirect.com/science/article/pii/S0166432815000169?via%3Dihub

Albert C Lo, V. C. (2010, October 14). *Reduction of freezing of gait in Parkinson's disease by repetitive robot-assisted treadmill training: a pilot study.* Retrieved from Journal of NeuroEngineering and Rehabilitation : https://link.springer.com/article/10.1186/1743-0003-7-51

Allan L. Adkin PhD James S. Frank PhD Mandar S. Jog MD, F. (2003, April 23). *Movement Disorders.* Retrieved from Wiley Online Library: https://onlinelibrary.wiley.com/doi/pdf/10.1002/mds.10396

Aman JE, E. N. (2015, January 28). *The effectiveness of proprioceptive training for improving motor function: a systematic review.* Retrieved from Frontiers in Human Neuro Science: https://www.ncbi.nlm.nih.gov/pubmed/25674059

An Bogaerts, C. D. (2009, May). *The Effect of Power Plate®Training on Cardiorespiratory Fitness and Muscle Strength in the Elderly.* Retrieved from Age and Ageing: https://powerplate.com/PowerPlate/media/powerplate/research/pdfs/the-effect-of-power-plate-training-on-cardiorespiratory-fitness-and-muscle-strength-in-the-elderly.pdf

Anat Mirelman, P. H.-E.-Y.-W.-P. (2016, October 6). *HHS Public Access, Arm Swing as a Potential New Prodromal Marker of Parkinson's Disease.* Retrieved from US National Library of Medicine, National Institute of Health: https://www.ncbi.nlm.nih.gov/pmc/articles/PMC5053872/

Anderson, D. B. (n.d.). *Premier Health of Summit.* Retrieved from Parkinson's Disease and Balance Disorders: https://www.drbriananderson.com/parkinsons-disease-balance-disorders/

Anneliese B. New, D. A. (2015, January 27). *The intrinsic resting state voice network in Parkinson's disease.* Retrieved from Human brain mapping: https://www.ncbi.nlm.nih.gov/pmc/articles/PMC4782783/

B.R.Bloem. (1992). *Postural instability in Parkinson's disease.* Retrieved from Clinical Neurology and Neurosurgery: https://www.sciencedirect.com/science/article/pii/030384679290018X

Barmore, D. R. (n.d.). *Conditions that Mimic Parkinson's.* Retrieved from Parkinson's Foundation: https://www.parkinson.org/Understanding-Parkinsons/Diagnosis/Conditions-that-Mimic-Parkinsons

Berg K, W.-D. S. (1992). Measuring balance in the elderly: validation of an instrument. *Can. J. Pub. Health*, S7-11.

Capecci M, S. C. (2014, February 5). *Postural rehabilitation and Kinesio taping for axial postural disorders in Parkinson's disease.* Retrieved from Arch Phys Med Rehabilitation: https://www.ncbi.nlm.nih.gov/pubmed/24508531

Carlijn D.J.M. Borm, a. K. (2019, May 23). *US National Library of Medicine* . Retrieved from Journal of Parkinson's Disease: https://www.ncbi.nlm.nih.gov/pmc/articles/PMC6597980/#ref001

Carlijn D.J.M. Borm, K. S. (2019, March 3). *The Neuro-Ophthalmological Assessment in Parkinson's Disease.* Retrieved from Journal of Parkinson's Disease: https://www.ncbi.nlm.nih.gov/pmc/articles/PMC6597980/#ref004

Charlotte Spay, G. M.-L. (2018, December 18). *Functional imaging correlates of akinesia in Parkinson's disease: Still open issues.* Retrieved from NeuroImage. Clinical: https://www.ncbi.nlm.nih.gov/pmc/articles/PMC6412010/

Christian T. Haasa, S. T. (2006, May 6). *The effects of random whole-body-vibration on motor symptoms in Parkinson's disease.* Retrieved from NeuroRehabilitation: https://content.iospress.com/download/neurorehabilitation/nre00299?id=neurorehabilitation%2Fnre00299

Clinic, C. (n.d.). *Othostatic Hypotension.* Retrieved from Cleveland Clinic: https://my.clevelandclinic.org/health/diseases/9385-orthostatic-hypotension

Clinic, M. (n.d.). *Restless legs syndrome.* Retrieved from Mayo Clinic: https://www.mayoclinic.org/diseases-conditions/restless-legs-syndrome/symptoms-causes/syc-20377168

da Silva Germanos S., V. B. (2019, June). *The impact of an aquatic exercise program on BDNF levels in Parkinson's disease patients:.* Retrieved from Functional Neurology: https://www.functionalneurology.com/common/php/portiere.php?ID=27768b8fee7b6635e76b53568e03c909

Den'etsu Sutoo, K. (2004, August 6). *Music improves dopaminergic neurotransmission: demonstration based on the effect of music on blood pressure regulation.* Retrieved from Brain Research: https://www.sciencedirect.com/science/article/abs/pii/S000689930400736X?via%3Dihub

Diagnosis – Rating Scales. (2017, March 8). Retrieved from Parkinsonsdisease.net: https://parkinsonsdisease.net/diagnosis/rating-scales-staging/

Dockx K, B. E. (2016). *Cochrane Library / Cochrane Database of Systematic Reviews.* Retrieved from Virtual reality for rehabilitation in Parkinson's disease (Review):

https://www.cochranelibrary.com/cdsr/doi/10.1002/14651858.CD010760.pu
b2/epdf/full

Elin Damsgård, R. C. (2007, July 4). *The Tampa Scale of Kinesiophobia: A Rasch analysis of its properties in subjects with low back and more widespread pain.* Retrieved from Journal of Rehabilitation Medicine: https://www.medicaljournals.se/jrm/content/html/10.2340/16501977-0125

Fahn, J. H. (2011). *Principles and Pratice of Movement Disorders, Second Edition.* Elsevier Saunders.

Fu R, L. X. (2016, May 10). *Clinical characteristics of fatigued Parkinson's patients and the response to dopaminergic treatment.* Retrieved from Translational Neurodegeneration: https://www.ncbi.nlm.nih.gov/pubmed/27175281

G C Pluck, R. G. (2002, December 1). *Apathy in Parkinson's disease.* Retrieved from Journal of Neurology, Neurosurgery, & Psychiatry: https://jnnp.bmj.com/content/73/6/636.full

Gray, P., & Hildebrand, K. (2000, August). *Fall Risk Factors in Parkinson's Disease.* Retrieved from Proquest: https://search.proquest.com/openview/d4db3059040cf223053d2cb1f307db73/1?pq-origsite=gscholar&cbl=48278

Guedes-Granzotti1, R. B. (2018, March). *Neuropsychomotor development and auditory development in preschool children.* Retrieved from Departamento de Fonoaudiologia da Universidade Federal de Sergipe : http://pepsic.bvsalud.org/pdf/rbcdh/v28n1/05.pdf

Hamm, T. (2017, December 13). *If You Want Different Results You Have To Try Different Approaches.* Retrieved from The Simple Dollar: https://www.thesimpledollar.com/if-you-want-different-results-you-have-to-try-different-approaches/

Huh YE1, H. S. (2016, February 3). *US National Library of Medicine National Institutes of Health.* Retrieved from PubMed: https://www.ncbi.nlm.nih.gov/pubmed/26883663

Ipatenco, S. (2018, November 16). *Parkour Facts.* Retrieved from SportsRec: https://www.sportsrec.com/7790983/parkour-facts

J M Senarda, S. R.-M. (1997). *Journal of Neurology, Neurosurgery, and Psychiatry.* Retrieved from

Prevalence of orthostatic hypotension in Parkinson's disease: https://jnnp.bmj.com/content/63/5/584.short

J. ANDREW BERKOWSKI, M. (2017, June 6). *Brain Health.* Retrieved from University of Michgan Health: https://healthblog.uofmhealth.org/brain-health/rem-sleep-behavior-disorder-parkinsons-disease-can-be-a-nightmare

Jennifer G. Goldman, B. A. (2018, July 26). *Cognitive impairment in Parkinson's disease: a report from a multidisciplinary symposium on unmet needs and future directions to maintain cognitive health*. Retrieved from NPJ Parkinson's Disease: https://www.ncbi.nlm.nih.gov/pmc/articles/PMC6018742/

Jennifer G. Goldman, M. M. (2015, August 1). *HHS Public Access, Premotor and non-motor features of Parkinson's disease*. Retrieved from US National Library of Medicine, National Institute of Health: https://www.ncbi.nlm.nih.gov/pmc/articles/PMC4181670/

John C. Murray, O. (n.d.). *Infinity Walk*. Retrieved from Murray Therapy: http://murraytherapy.com/activities/infinity-walk

John J Ratey, M. (2008). *Spark.* New York, NY: Little, Brown and Company.

John J. Ratey, M. (2014). *Go Wild.* New York, NY: Little, Brown and Company.

Josefa M. Domingos, a. C. (2015, September 14). *US National Library of Medicine* . Retrieved from Journal of Parkinson's Disease: https://www.ncbi.nlm.nih.gov/pmc/articles/PMC4923751/

Jost, W. H. (2013, April). *Urological problems in Parkinson's disease: clinical aspects*. Retrieved from Journal of Neural Transmission: https://link.springer.com/article/10.1007/s00702-012-0914-8

Juliette H Lanskey, P. M.-C. (2018, September). *Can neuroimaging predict dementia in Parkinson's disease?* Retrieved from Oxford Academic / Brain / A Journal of Neurology: https://academic.oup.com/brain/article/141/9/2545/5078251

Karen Frei, D. D. (2017, March 15). *Hallucinations and the spectrum of psychosis in Parkinson's disease*. Retrieved from Journal of the Neurological Sciences: https://www.jns-journal.com/article/S0022-510X(17)30013-8/abstract

Koller WC1, G. S.-O. (1989, April 12). *US National Library of Medicine National Institutes of Health*. Retrieved from www.ncbi.nlm.nih.gov: https://www.ncbi.nlm.nih.gov/pubmed/2720700

Lang, D. A. (2018, October 4). *New Developments & Future Treatments in PD - Dr. Anthony Lang - UF Parkinson Symposium 2018*. Retrieved from https://www.youtube.com/user/UniversityofFlorida: https://www.youtube.com/watch?v=Y9S-6jv3ivE&t=1481s

Laura B. Zahodne, M. D. (2011, April 25). *The Case for Testing Memory with Both Stories and Word Lists Prior to DBS Surgery for Parkinson's Disease*. Retrieved from US National Library of Medicine /National Institute of Health:

https://www.ncbi.nlm.nih.gov/pmc/articles/PMC3077807/

Leland E Dibble, P. P. (2016, April 1). *EXERCISE AND MEDICATION EFFECTS ON PERSONS WITH PARKINSON DISEASE ACROSS THE*

DOMAINS OF DISABILITY: A RANDOMIZED CLINICAL TRIAL.
Retrieved from Journal of neurologic physical therapy:
https://www.ncbi.nlm.nih.gov/pmc/articles/PMC4366306/
Lexico. (n.d.). *Lexico.* Retrieved from Lexico:
https://www.lexico.com/en/definition/visuospatial
Life, T. f. (n.d.). *Fascial Movement Taping.* Retrieved from Thrive for Life:
https://thrive4lifenow.com/fascial-movement-taping-fmt/
Linlin Gao, 1. J. (2017, March 30). *US National Library of Medicine .*
Retrieved from Scientific Reports:
https://www.ncbi.nlm.nih.gov/pmc/articles/PMC5372469/
Lynda Elaine Powell, A. M. (1995, January 1). *The Activities-specific
Balance Confidence (ABC) Scale.* Retrieved from The Journals of
Gerontology: https://academic.oup.com/biomedgerontology/article-
abstract/50A/1/M28/616764
M Samuel, M. R.-O. (2015, January 1). *Impulse Control Disorders in
Parkinson's Disease:Management, Controversies, and Potential
Approaches.* Retrieved from US National Library of Medicine, National
Institutes of Health:
https://www.ncbi.nlm.nih.gov/pmc/articles/PMC5077247/
M.J. de Dreua, A. d. (2011, December 10). *Rehabilitation, exercise therapy
and music in patients with Parkinson's disease: a meta-analysis of the effects
of music-based movement therapy on walking ability, balance and quality of
life.* Retrieved from Parkinsonism & Related Disorders:
https://www.sciencedirect.com/science/article/abs/pii/S1353802011700360
Machteld Roelants, S. V. (2004, June). *Power Plate® training Increases
Knee-Extension Strength and Speed of Movement in Older Women.*
Retrieved from Journal of the American Geriatrics Society:
https://powerplate.com/PowerPlate/media/powerplate/research/pdfs/power-
plate-training-proves-effective-for-the-elderly.pdf
Merzenich, D. M. (2013). *Soft-Wired.* San Francisco: Parnassus Publishing,
LLC.
Michelle E. Fullard, J. F. (2017, August 22). *Springer Neuroscience Bulletin,
Olfactory Dysfunction as an Early Biomarker in Parkinson's Disease.*
Retrieved from US National Library of Medicine National Institue of Health:
https://www.ncbi.nlm.nih.gov/pmc/articles/PMC5636737/
Michelle R. Ciucci, P. C.-S.-S.-N. (2015, June 23). *Early Identification and
Treatment of Communication and Swallowing Deficits in Parkinson Disease.*
Retrieved from Ciucci, Michelle R et al. "Early identification and treatment
of communication and swallowing deficits in Parkinson disease." Seminars
in speech and language vol. 34,3 (2013): 185-202. doi:10.1055/s-0033-
1358367: https://www.ncbi.nlm.nih.gov/pmc/articles/PMC4477682/

MoCA. (n.d.). *Montreal Cognitive Assessment*. Retrieved from Montreal
Cognitive Assessment: https://www.mocatest.org/the-moca-test/

Murat Emre MD, D. A. (2007, May 31). *Clinical diagnostic criteria for
dementia associated with Parkinson's disease*. Retrieved from Movement
Disorders: https://onlinelibrary.wiley.com/doi/full/10.1002/mds.21507

Norman Doidge, M. (2007). *The Brain that Changes Itself*. New York, N.Y.:
Penguin Group.

Norman Doidge, M. (2016). *The Brain's Way of Healing*. New York, NY:
Peguin Random House.

Olivia E. Knowles, E. J. (2018, September). *Inadequate sleep and muscle
strength: Implications for resistance training*. Retrieved from Journal of
Science and Medicine in Sport:
https://www.sciencedirect.com/science/article/abs/pii/S1440244018300306

Pablo Martinez-Martin, J. M.-A.-B. (2017, March 15). *Distribution and
impact on quality of life of the pain modalities assessed by the King's
Parkinson's disease pain scale*. Retrieved from Martinez-Martin, P., Manuel
Rojo-Abuin, J., Rizos, A., Rodriguez-Blazquez, C., Trenkwalder, C.,
Perkins, L., ... KPPS, EUROPAR and the IPMDS Non Motor PD Study
Group (2017). Distribution and impact on quality of life of the pain
modalities assessed by the K:
https://www.ncbi.nlm.nih.gov/pmc/articles/PMC5459857/

Pacchetti, C. M., Mancini, F. M., Aglieri, R., Fundarò, C. M., Martignoni, E.
M., & Nappi, G. M. (2000, May-June). *Active Music Therapy in Parkinson's
Disease: An Integrative Method for Motor and Emotional Rehabilitation*.
Retrieved from Psychosomatic Medicine:
https://journals.lww.com/psychosomaticmedicine/Abstract/2000/05000/Acti
ve_Music_Therapy_in_Parkinson_s_Disease__An.12.aspx

Pacchetti, C. M., Mancini, F. M., Aglieri, R., Fundarò, C. M., Martignoni, E.
M., & Nappi, G. M. (2000, May-June). *Active Music Therapy in Parkinson's
Disease: An Integrative Method for Motor and Emotional Rehabilitation*.
Retrieved from Psychosomatic Medicine:
https://journals.lww.com/psychosomaticmedicine/Abstract/2000/05000/Acti
ve_Music_Therapy_in_Parkinson_s_Disease__An.12.aspx

Physio-Pedia. (n.d.). *Berg Balance Scale with Instructions*. Retrieved from
Physio-pedia.com: https://www.physio-
pedia.com/images/b/bd/Berg_balance_scale_with_instructions.pdf

Plate, P. (n.d.). *Research*. Retrieved from Power Plate:
https://powerplate.com/education-and-training/medical-rehab

Powell, S. (2014, May 16). *Proven Powerful Health Benefits of Power Plate*.
Retrieved from Fitness Superstore Blog: https://www.fitness-
superstore.co.uk/blog/guest-blog-11-proven-powerful-health-benefits-of-
power-plate/

Priti Gros, M. a. (2018, September 1). *SLEEP AND CIRCADIAN RHYTHM DISORDERS IN PARKINSON'S DISEASE.* Retrieved from US National Library of

Medicine, National Institute of Health: https://www.ncbi.nlm.nih.gov/pmc/articles/PMC5699506/

Quinsey, A. (2017, May 8). *What is Spatial Awareness and why is it important to children?* Retrieved from ModulePlay Commercial Systems: https://www.moduplay.com.au/spatial-awareness-important-children/

Rudzińska M, B. S.-P. (2013, October). *US National Library of Medicine National Institutes of Health.* Retrieved from PubMed: https://www.ncbi.nlm.nih.gov/pubmed/24166563

Rudzińska M1, M. M. (2007, October). *Falls in different types of Parkinson's disease.* Retrieved from US National Library of Medicine National Institutes of Health: https://www.ncbi.nlm.nih.gov/pubmed/18033639

Sakata, K. (2014, January 27). *Brain-Derived Neurotrophic Factor for Depression Therapeutics.* Retrieved from Austin Publishing Group: https://austinpublishinggroup.com/pharmacology-therapeutics/fulltext/ajpt-v2-id1006.php

Sharareh Sharififar, P. R. (2014, July). *The Effects of Whole Body Vibration on Mobility and Balance in Parkinson Disease: a Systematic Review.* Retrieved from Iranian Journal of Medicine Sciences: https://www.ncbi.nlm.nih.gov/pmc/articles/PMC4100042/

Sharon L. Tennstedt, P. a. (2015, February 25). *The ACTIVE Study: Study Overview and Major Findings.* Retrieved from Journal of Aging and Health: https://www.ncbi.nlm.nih.gov/pmc/articles/PMC3934012/?fbclid=IwAR2S2HG35_ht6WMpj53-O2neaa8VAlDq4nsNUgzlo2D_VlwMC1JhnUYxk98

Shill H, S. M. (2002, June 23). *Respiratory complications of Parkinson's disease.* Retrieved from Thieme: https://www.thieme-connect.com/products/ejournals/abstract/10.1055/s-2002-33034

Silvia Marazzi, P. K. (2020, January 14). *beneficial effects on balance stability and mobility in individuals with Parkinson disease.* Retrieved from European Journal of Physical and Rehanbilitation Medicine: https://www.minervamedica.it/en/journals/europa-medicophysica/article.php?cod=R33Y9999N00A20011406

Şimşek TT1, T. B. (2011, March 11). *The effects of Kinesio® taping on sitting posture, functional independence and gross motor function in children with cerebral palsy.* Retrieved from Disability and Rehabilitation: https://www.ncbi.nlm.nih.gov/pubmed/21401336

Sinai, C. (n.d.). *Diagnosing Parkinson's Disease.* Retrieved from Cedars Sinai: https://www.cedars-sinai.edu/Patients/Programs-and-

Services/Imaging-Center/For-Patients/Exams-by-Procedure/Nuclear-Medicine/DatScan/

Tan, T. P.-K. (2012, February 27). *Linking restless legs syndrome with Parkinson's disease: clinical, imaging and genetic evidence*. Retrieved from US National Library of Medicine National Institute of Health: https://www.ncbi.nlm.nih.gov/pmc/articles/PMC3514082/

Tao Wu, M. H. (2017, August 21). *Motor automaticity in Parkinson's disease*. Retrieved from Neurobiology of disease: https://www.ncbi.nlm.nih.gov/pmc/articles/PMC5565272/

Thedon T, M. K. (2011, March 31). *Degraded postural performance after muscle fatigue can be compensated by skin stimulation*. Retrieved from Gait and Posture: https://www.ncbi.nlm.nih.gov/pubmed/21454076

Tie-mei Zhang, M. S.-y.-s.-j.-h.-d.-j. (2016, December 16). *Nonmotor symptoms in patients with Parkinson disease*. Retrieved from Medicine (Baltimore): https://www.ncbi.nlm.nih.gov/pmc/articles/PMC5268024/

Unknown. (n.d.). *COGNITIVE MEASURES* . Retrieved from Niagenetics Initiative: http://niageneticsinitiative.org/procedures/PDF/Sections/LOAD_Cognitive_Measures_2006.pdf

unknown. (n.d.). *Memory and Levels of Explanation*. Retrieved from Mental Construction: https://www.mentalconstruction.com/memory-levels-explanation/

van Wamelen DJ, L. V.-M. (2019, April 17). *Exploring hyperhidrosis and related thermoregulatory symptoms as a possible clinical identifier for the dysautonomic subtype of Parkinson's disease*. Retrieved from Journal of Neurology: https://www.ncbi.nlm.nih.gov/pubmed/30997572

Vera Bittner, S. S. (n.d.). *The 6 Minute Walk Test*. Retrieved from Cardiology Advisor: https://www.thecardiologyadvisor.com/home/decision-support-in-medicine/cardiology/the-6-minute-walk-test/

Waddell G, N. M. (1993, February). *A Fear-Avoidance Beliefs Questionnaire (FABQ) and the role of fear-avoidance beliefs in chronic low back pain and disability*. Retrieved from Pain: https://www.ncbi.nlm.nih.gov/pubmed/8455963

Made in the USA
Middletown, DE
04 December 2022